T0222591

Lecture Notes in Computer Science   **8680**

More information about this series at http://www.springer.com/series/7412

Marius George Linguraru · Cristina Oyarzun Laura
Raj Shekhar · Stefan Wesarg
Miguel Ángel González Ballester · Klaus Drechsler
Yoshinobu Sato · Marius Erdt (Eds.)

Clinical Image-Based Procedures

Translational Research in Medical Imaging

Third International Workshop, CLIP 2014
Held in Conjunction with MICCAI 2014
Boston, MA, USA, September 14, 2014
Revised Selected Papers

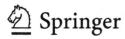 Springer

Editors

Marius George Linguraru
Children's National Health System
Washington, DC
USA

Cristina Oyarzun Laura
Fraunhofer IGD
Darmstadt
Germany

Raj Shekhar
Children's National Health System
Washington, DC
USA

Stefan Wesarg
Fraunhofer IGD
Darmstadt
Germany

Miguel Ángel González Ballester
ICREA - Universitat Pompeu Fabra
Barcelona
Spain

Klaus Drechsler
Fraunhofer IGD
Darmstadt
Germany

Yoshinobu Sato
Nara Institute of Science and Technology
   (NAIST)
Ikoma, Nara
Japan

Marius Erdt
Fraunhofer IDM@NTU
Singapore
Singapore

ISSN 0302-9743   ISSN 1611-3349   (electronic)
Lecture Notes in Computer Science
ISBN 978-3-319-13908-1   ISBN 978-3-319-13909-8   (eBook)
DOI 10.1007/978-3-319-13909-8

Library of Congress Control Number: 2014958153

LNCS Sublibrary: SL6 – Image Processing, Computer Vision, Pattern Recognition, and Graphics

Springer International Publishing AG Switzerland is part of Springer Science+Business Media
(www.springer.com)

Preface

On September 14, 2014, The Third International Workshop on Clinical Image based Procedures: Translational Research in Medical Imaging (CLIP 2014) was held in Boston, MA, USA in conjunction with the International Conference on Medical Image Computing and Computer Assisted Intervention (MICCAI 2014). The successful meeting was a productive and exciting forum for the discussion and dissemination of clinical applications of medical imaging, state-of-the-art methods for image-based planning, and development and evaluation of new medical procedures and therapies. The workshop was co-organized by Childrens National Health System, Fraunhofer IGD and IDM@NTU, Nara Institute of Science and Technology, and Universitat Pompeu Fabra.

Over the past few years, there has been a considerable and growing interest in the development and evaluation of new translational image-based techniques in the modern hospital. For a decade or more, the outstanding proliferation of medical image applications has created a need for greater study and scrutiny of the clinical application and validation of such methods. New strategies are essential to ensure a smooth and effective translation of computational image-based techniques into the clinic. For these reasons and to complement other technology focused MICCAI workshops on computer-assisted interventions, CLIP's major focus was on translational research filling the gaps between basic science and clinical applications.

A highlight of the workshop was the subject of strategies for personalized medicine to enhance diagnosis, treatment, and interventions. Members of the medical imaging community were encouraged to submit work centered on specific clinical applications, including techniques and procedures based on comprehensive clinical image data or already in use and evaluated by clinical users. The event brought together over 40 world-class researchers and clinicians who presented ways to strengthen links between computer scientists and engineers, and surgeons, interventional radiologists, and radiation oncologists.

In the tradition of our previous workshops, CLIP 2014 was a successful venue for the dissemination of emerging image-based clinical techniques, the analysis of the current uptake of advanced computational imaging techniques, and the discussion of the main hurdles for their clinical translation and how to overcome them. Specific topics included pre-interventional image segmentation and classification (to support diagnosis and clinical decision making), shape analysis for anatomical modeling, interventional and surgical planning and analysis of dynamic images, and evaluation, visualization, and simulation techniques for image based procedures. Clinical applications covered brain diseases, cardiac defects, orthopedics, inflammatory diseases, blood vessels, cochlear defects, and cancer of the head and neck, breast, prostate, and lung in adults and children. During two keynote sessions, clinical highlights were presented and discussed by Pedro del Nido, MD, Chairman of the Department of Cardiovascular Surgery at Boston Children's Hospital and William E. Ladd Professor of Child Surgery at Harvard Medical School (minimally invasive robotic surgery on the beating heart), and Thomas Bortfeld, PhD, Director of the Physics Division at Massachusetts General Hospital and Professor in the Department of Radiation Oncology at Harvard Medical School (imaging radiation and proton therapy). We are grateful to our keynote speakers for their compelling presentations and vibrant participation in workshop discussions.

In response to the call for papers, 26 original manuscripts were submitted for presentation at CLIP 2014. Each of the manuscripts underwent a meticulous double-blind peer review by a minimum of two members of the Program Committee, prestigious experts in the field of medical image analysis and clinical translations of technology. Seventy-three percent or 19 of the manuscripts were accepted for presentation at the workshop: 12 or 46 % as long oral presentations, and 7 as short oral and poster contributions. Contributors represented three continents: Europe, North America, and Asia. The six papers with the highest review score were nominated to be considered as best papers. From them, the three best papers were chosen by votes cast by workshop participants who had attended all six presentations of the nominated papers (workshop organizers excepted). As a result, three awards were presented. The first place went to Juan Cerrolaza, Sergio Vera, Alexis Bagué, Mario Ceresa, Pablo Migliorelli, Marius George Linguraru, and Miguel Ángel González Ballester from Children's National Health System in Washington, DC, USA, and Alma IT Systems and Universitat Pompeu Fabra in Barcelona, Spain for their work in shape modeling of the cochlea and surrounding risk structures for minimally invasive cochlear implant surgery. The second place was presented to Amit Shah, Oliver Zettinig, Tobias Maurer, Cristina Precup, Christian Schulte zu Berge, Jakob Weiss, Benjamin Frisch, Nassir Navab from Technische Universität München in Germany for their advancements on multimodal image-guided prostate biopsy. The third place was conferred on Nishant Uniyal, Farhad Imani, Amir Tahmasebi, Peter Choyke, Baris Turkbey, Peter Pinto, Bradford Wood, Sheng Xu, Jin Tae Kwak, Pingkun Yan, Jochen Kruecker, Shyam Bharat, Harsh Agarwal, Purang Abolmaesumi, Parvin Mousavi, Mehdi Moradi from University of British Columbia, Vancouver, BC, Canada, Queen's University, Kingston, ON, Canada, Philips Research North America, Briarcliff Manor, NY, USA, and National Institutes of Health, Bethesda, MD, USA for their contributions to ultrasound-based predication of prostate cancer in MRI-guided biopsy. We would like to congratulate warmly all the prize winners for their outstanding work and exciting presentations and thank our sponsors, EXOCAD and MedCom, and HEAR-EU for their support.

We would also like to acknowledge the invaluable contributions of our entire Program Committee without whose assistance CLIP 2014 would not have been as successful and stimulating. Our thanks also go to all the authors in this volume for the high quality of their work and the commitment of time and effort. Finally, we are grateful to the MICCAI 2014 organizers, and particularly Polina Golland, Nobuhiko Hata, Georg Langs, Mehdi Moradi, Sonia Pujol, and Martin Styner, for supporting the organization of CLIP 2014.

October 2014

Marius George Linguraru
Cristina Oyarzun Laura
Raj Shekhar
Stefan Wesarg
Miguel Ángel González Ballester
Klaus Drechsler
Yoshinobu Sato
Marius Erdt

Organization

Committees

Organizing Committee

Klaus Drechsler	Fraunhofer IGD, Germany
Marius Erdt	Fraunhofer IDM@NTU, Singapore
Marius George Linguraru	Children's National Health System, USA
Miguel Ángel González Ballester	ICREA - Universitat Pompeu Fabra, Spain
Cristina Oyarzun Laura	Fraunhofer IGD, Germany
Yoshinobu Sato	Nara Institute of Science and Technology, Japan
Raj Shekhar	Children's National Health System, USA
Stefan Wesarg	Fraunhofer IGD, Germany

Program Committee

Jorge Bernal	Universitat Autonoma de Barcelona, Spain
Mario Ceresa	Pompeu Fabra University, Spain
Juan Cerrolaza	Children's National Health System, USA
Xinjian Chen	Soochow University, China
Yufei Chen	Tongji University, China
Thiago dos Santos	SENAI Institute of Innovation in Embedded Systems, Brazil
Jan Egger	TU Graz, Austria
Wissam El Hakimi	TU Darmstadt, Germany
Gloria Fernández Esparrach	Hospital Clinic Barcelona, Spain
Moti Freimann	Harvard Medical School, USA
Debora Gil	Universitat Autonoma de Barcelona, Spain
Enrico Grisan	University of Padova, Italy
Tobias Heimann	Siemens, Germany
Xin Kang	Siemens, China
Michael Kelm	Siemens, Germany
Jianfei Liu	Duke University, USA
Xinyang Liu	Children's National Health System, USA
Yoshitaka Masutani	Hiroshima City University, Japan
Diana Nabers	German Cancer Research Center, Germany
Danielle Pace	Massachussets Institute of Technology, USA
Mauricio Reyes	University of Bern, Switzerland
Akinobu Shimizu	Tokyo University of Agriculture and Technology, Japan
Ronald M. Summers	National Institutes of Health, USA
Kenji Suzuki	University of Chicago, USA
Zeike Taylor	University of Sheffield, UK

Shijun Wang	National Institutes of Health, USA
Thomas Wittenberg	Fraunhofer IIS, Germany
Ziv Yaniv	Children's National Health System, USA
Qian Zhao	Children's National Health System, USA
Stephan Zidowitz	Fraunhofer MEVIS, Germany

Sponsoring Institutions

exocad GmbH
HEAR-EU Project
MedCom GmbH

Contents

An Open Source Multimodal Image-Guided Prostate Biopsy Framework

Amit Shah[1]([✉]), Oliver Zettinig[1], Tobias Maurer[2], Cristina Precup[1],
Christian Schulte zu Berge[1], Jakob Weiss[1], Benjamin Frisch[1],
and Nassir Navab[1]

[1] Computer Aided Medical Procedures,
Technische Universität München, Munich, Germany
amit.shah@tum.de
[2] Poliklinik und Klinik für Urologie, Klinikum Rechts der Isar,
Technische Universität München, Munich, Germany

Abstract. Although various modalities are used in prostate cancer imaging, transrectal ultrasound (TRUS) guided biopsy remains the gold standard for diagnosis. However, TRUS suffers from low sensitivity, leading to an elevated rate of false negative results. Magnetic Resonance Imaging (MRI) on the other hand provides currently the most accurate image-based evaluation of the prostate. Thus, TRUS/MRI fusion image-guided biopsy has evolved to be the method of choice to circumvent the limitations of TRUS-only biopsy. Most commercial frameworks that offer such a solution rely on rigid TRUS/MRI fusion and rarely use additional information from other modalities such as Positron Emission Tomography (PET). Other frameworks require long interaction times and are complex to integrate with the clinical workflow. Available solutions are not fully able to meet the clinical requirements of speed and high precision at low cost simultaneously. We introduce an open source fusion biopsy framework that is low cost, simple to use and has minimal overhead in clinical workflow. Hence, it is ideal as a research platform for the implementation and rapid bench to bedside translation of new image registration and visualization approaches. We present the current status of the framework that uses pre-interventional PET and MRI rigidly registered with 3D TRUS for prostate biopsy guidance and discuss results from first clinical cases.

Keywords: Prostate cancer · Multimodal image-guided biopsy · PET · MRI · TRUS · Open source software

1 Introduction

Prostate cancer is one of the most common cancers worldwide [1]. However, survival rates are high if it is diagnosed early and treated on time. The gold standard to confirm prostate cancer is transrectal ultrasound (TRUS) guided systematic 10–12 core biopsy. Although TRUS provides real-time anatomical guidance, its sensitivity for prostate cancer is rather low. Hence, TRUS guided

M.G. Linguraru et al. (Eds.): CLIP 2014, LNCS 8680, pp. 1–8, 2014.
DOI: 10.1007/978-3-319-13909-8_1

systematic biopsies may miss important cancer sites [12]. On the other hand, multi-parametric MRI and PET have higher cancer detection rate as reported in the studies presented in the review paper by Turkbey et al. [12]. Further studies [3,6,10] have shown that TRUS/MRI fusion image-guided targeted biopsy might detect significantly more malignant lesions compared to using TRUS alone.

Many urology clinics have access to advanced imaging modalities such as CT, MRI or nuclear medicine and an increasing number of urologists performs cognitive fusion of these multimodal images while performing TRUS guided biopsy. However, cognitive fusion is prone to human error and does not improve the results significantly as presented by Delongchamps et al. [3]. Hence, automatic fusion of pre-interventional imaging, especially of MRI and PET with TRUS, is highly desired.

Literature Review. One challenge lies in combining pre-interventional multimodal images with interventional TRUS automatically, with acceptable accuracy and without exceeding the permissible time limits of the clinical workflow. Efforts towards TRUS/MRI registration are summarized by Sperling et al. [10]. While classical approaches mostly rely on either surface based or extracted fiducial driven algorithms, more recent approaches attempt deformable registration based on prostate surface models using spline basis functions [7] or on probabilistic and statistical shape models [9]. These algorithms rely on the manual segmentation of prostate surfaces which requires an extended interaction of the physician, which makes it difficult to integrate into the clinical routine.

A further challenge is the development of a biopsy system that uses such fusion images for guidance. Commercial solutions come each with their drawbacks, reducing their acceptance in urological routine. Most systems use 2D TRUS probes and track their position to compound a 3D TRUS image. Percu-Nav (Philips, NL) and Hi-RVS (Hitachi, JP) both use electromagnetic tracking, subject to disturbances of the electromagnetic field and ensuing low tracking accuracy. Artemis (Eigen, US) requires a mechanical arm to record the position of the US probe and does surface based TRUS/MRI elastic registration. The BioJET (GeoScan, USA) and BiopSee (Medcom, DE) systems both mount the US probe on a stepper to acquire information about the position of the US probe. To our knowledge, only the Koelis system (Uronav, France) avoids the challenges of a tracking system by using a 3D TRUS probe. It uses elastic registration algorithms but requires TRUS/TRUS registration as an intermediate step for TRUS/MRI registration.

Until recently, PET/TRUS fusion for prostate biopsy has generated only moderate interest mainly due to the low specificity of currently available tracers like ^{11}C-acetate, ^{11}C-choline and ^{18}F-FDG [12]. However, with the introduction of ^{68}Ga labelled ligands of Prostate Specific Membrane Antigen (PSMA), PET/TRUS fusion might gain increasing attention [4].

Proposed Solution. In this work, we propose a solution that leverages the use of open source software to develop a multimodal image-guided system for transrectal prostate biopsy that combines pre-interventional PET-MRI with interventional 3D TRUS. This low cost approach aims at providing a research platform for the implementation and rapid translation into clinical use of new image registration and visualisation approaches. We use the PLUS framework [5] for ultrasound probe calibration, tracked image acquisition and volume reconstruction. PLUS requires further packages such as ITK for image processing [14], VTK for visualization [8] and OpenIGTLink [11] for communication with other systems. Our application is developed using CAMPVis [2], an open source visualization framework from our group, that offers image registration and real-time slice rendering based on tracking information.

The software components and the targeted biopsy system are explained in Sect. 2. The outcomes of first clinical cases using rigid landmark-based registration are presented in Sect. 3. The conclusion and future work are outlined in Sect. 4.

2   Method

2.1   System Setup

Our system, illustrated in Fig. 1, is lightweight in terms of workflow and resources. It consists of a conventional ultrasound system, optical tracking and a workstation. The ultrasound system is a Hitachi AVIUS with a front fire trans-rectal probe that provides 2D ultrasound images. The ultrasound probe is tracked by an NDI Polaris® optical tracking system. Since we do not have direct access to RF data from the ultrasound machine, we use a frame grabber to acquire high resolution 1280×1024 digital images. The workstation has 2 Intel Xeon® processors running at 2.13 GHz with 32 GB RAM and a NVIDIA GeForce® 8800 GTS 512 Graphics card. The 3D TRUS image acquisition and biopsy guidance are based on PLUS and CAMPVis respectively, both are open source software frameworks for medical applications.

2.2   Clinical Protocol

The 3D TRUS acquisition and PET-MRI-TRUS registration procedure were easily integrated into the existing clinical workflow without much overhead in time or effort. Figure 2 shows the steps in the multimodal image-guided prostate biopsy. The system has already been used for biopsies of two patients, after obtaining their informed consent.

3D TRUS Acquisition Using PLUS. The first step in the fusion image-guided biopsy procedure is to acquire a 3D TRUS volume. This requires the spatial calibration of the ultrasound probe, a tracked ultrasound acquisition and reconstruction of the 3D volume from 2D ultrasound slices. All these steps are performed as per the methods given in Lasso et al. in [5].

Temporal and Spatial Calibration. An optical target, tracked by the optical tracking system (transformation $^{probe}T_{world}$), is mounted on the shaft of the front fire TRUS probe, opposite of the biopsy needle guide. The ultrasound images are

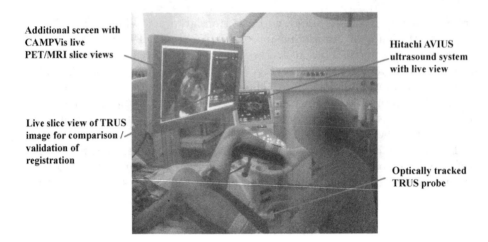

Additional screen with
CAMPVis live
PET/MRI slice views

Hitachi AVIUS
ultrasound system
with live view

Live slice view of TRUS
image for comparison /
validation of
registration

Optically tracked
TRUS probe

Fig. 1. Urologist performing prostate biopsy using multimodal image guidance.

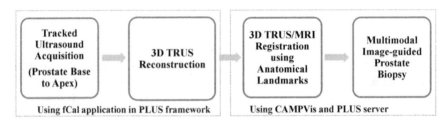

Fig. 2. Overview of the clinical procedure for multimodal image-guided prostate biopsy.

acquired in a high resolution digital format at 30 fps using a frame grabber card. This maintains compatibility to other ultrasound systems. Temporal calibration is done to account for any time lag between the tracking and the video frame. The spatial transformation $^{frame}T_{probe}$ between the image frame origin and the optical target is found using fCal application and a 3N-wire phantom provided in PLUS. It should be noted that this calibration procedure has to be performed only once as long as the target is fixed to the probe and the ultrasound image parameters, such as depth and focus, remain constant.

Tracked Ultrasound and Compounding. Another optical target, which acts as a reference (transformation $^{ref}T_{world}$), is attached to the biopsy chair where the patient is positioned in the lithotomy position. Using fCal, tracked ultrasound frames are continuously recorded while the urologist manually moves the probe from the prostate base to the apex. Applying a forward warping technique, the tracked frames are then compounded into a 3D TRUS volume. Hereby, the transformation $^{ref}T_{chair}$ between the reference target and the standard axes of the chair allows to align the 3D TRUS axes according to the DICOM standard, in order to preposition the volumes for subsequent registration. Figure 3 shows

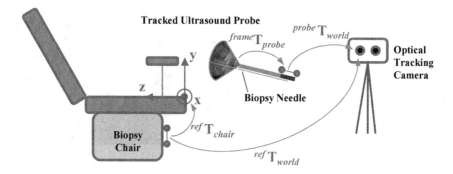

Fig. 3. Schematic setup, illustrating coordinate systems and transformations.

all transformations mentioned in Eq. 1:

$$^{frame}T_{3DTRUS} = {}^{ref}T_{chair} \cdot ({}^{ref}T_{world})^{-1} \cdot {}^{probe}T_{world} \cdot {}^{frame}T_{probe} \quad (1)$$

Landmark-Based Image Registration in CAMPVis. In order to align the MRI and acquired 3D TRUS volumes, a landmark-based image registration is performed. To that end, axial, coronal or sagittal slices of both images are presented in CAMPVis next to each other, allowing the urologist to select four corresponding anatomical landmarks by mouse clicks. Employing the Umeyama method [13], the rigid transformation $^{MRI}T_{3DTRUS}$ is solved and a fused image is presented to the physician. As PET and MRI volumes are acquired with a Siemens integrated wholebody PET-MRI scanner, they are intrinsically registered to each other, facilitating a transfer of lesions from PET to MRI images as shown in Fig. 4. As a result, the multimodal image registration is quickly achieved and can be performed in clinical routine without interrupting the procedure, during the preparation of local anesthesia.

Tracking and Navigation for Biopsy Guidance. The final step of the procedure is a targeted biopsy under multimodal image guidance. Apart from the 2D live ultrasound image shown on the screen of the ultrasound scanner, our framework provides the urologist in real time with corresponding slice views of one or more pre-operative images such as PET or MRI (cf. Fig. 1). In CAMPVis, the correct slicing planes are determined by the x- and y-axes of the following coordinate system:

$$^{frame}T_{MRI} = ({}^{MRI}T_{3DTRUS})^{-1} \cdot {}^{frame}T_{3DTRUS} \quad (2)$$

For the computation of $^{frame}T_{3DTRUS}$, only the current tracked positions of the ultrasound probe and the reference target need to be updated, which is achieved by forwarding tracking information from the PLUS server over the OpenIGTLink protocol. For navigation, a virtual biopsy guide that indicates an approximate needle insertion path is provided by the ultrasound machine and shown on the live ultrasound image. The urologist maneuvers the probe such that the virtual biopsy guide aligns with the target and biopsies are taken.

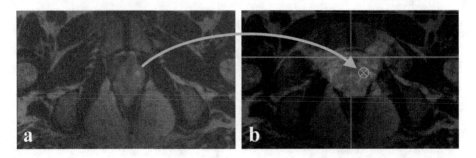

Fig. 4. Transfer of biopsy targets from PET to 3D TRUS via MRI for patient case 1. **(a)** PET/MRI with targets in pink, **(b)** 3D TRUS (green) registered to MRI image (red) after landmark-based registration (Color figure online).

3   Results

The first prototype of this platform was assessed in two patients, after they gave their informed consent, by an experienced urologist as per the workflow in Fig. 2. These patients had a clinical suspicion of prostate cancer but previously negative biopsy results. Hence, the patients underwent PET-MRI examination before the biopsy procedure. Figure 1 shows the system setup in our urology clinic during the fusion biopsy procedure.

System Performance. The time taken for the 3D TRUS acquisition and TRUS/ MRI registration was less than 10 min in both clinical cases. The tracked ultrasound acquisition is done during a routine US prostate examination that precedes every biopsy. The registration is performed in less than 5 min while the patient is waiting for the local anaesthesia to take effect. Thus, there is not much overhead in time as compared to conventional TRUS-guided systematic prostate biopsy. Figure 4(a) shows the PET-MRI image of patient number 1 for the identification of targets for biopsy. Figure 4(b) shows the TRUS/MRI fusion image after anatomical landmark-based registration for the same patient.

Clinical Cases. The clinical cases of two patients are summarized in Table 1. In both cases, the MRI was equivocal and the PET image revealed suspicious regions.

Table 1. Overview of clinical data and results using proposed targeted biopsy system.

Case	PSA value (ng/ml)	Targeted biopsy	Histology results
1	5.4	2	Prostate carcinoma left apical
2	7.5	2	No malignancy

Case 1 was a 45 year-old patient, *status post* a previous prostate biopsy one year ago with no malignancies found. With a rising PSA value of currently

5.4 ng/ml, the ^{68}Ga PSMA PET-MRI showed a highly suspicious area in the left apical central zone. For the systematic biopsy (10 cores), histology examination identified prostate carcinoma with a Gleason score of 6 in the left apical and the left central region of the prostate. The two targeted biopsy samples were also tested positive in histology, confirming a prostate carcinoma in the left apical site. Therefore, our system was able to identify, map and target the suspicious region for prostate cancer diagnosis.

Case 2 was a 58 year-old patient. Similarly to case 1, no malignancies had been identified in a previous prostate biopsy. Due to a rising PSA value of currently 7.5 ng/ml, the patient underwent ^{68}Ga PSMA PET-MRI, which showed only a slight expression of PSMA in the median peripheral zone on both sides and a moderate suspicion of prostate cancer. Histology results were negative for both the 10-core systematic biopsy and the 2-core targeted biopsy.

4 Conclusion

We presented a fusion image-guided system for targeted prostate biopsy based on open source software. We presented preliminary clinical results in two patients. We used PET-MRI images registered with 3D TRUS to identify, map and guide the biopsy. The time and resource overhead for the entire procedure compared to the conventional biopsy routine was minimal.

This open source software solution has many advantages that makes it ideal as a research platform. It is extremely useful for translational clinical research and can serve as a test bench to evaluate the medical impact of new developments. It further offers flexibility to modify or extend the software applications and community support for the development. The code sharing helps for rapid development and prevents duplicating research efforts. The overall system cost is significantly reduced compared to commercially available systems. Translating this prototype into a fully clinically acceptable solution will require further efforts.

We will extend the framework with advanced registration and visualisation algorithms that may further simplify the procedure and increase the precision in targeted biopsy.

Acknowledgments. This work is partially supported by the EU 7th Framework Program projects Marie Curie Early Initial Training Network Fellowship (PITN-GA-2011-289355-PicoSEC-MCNet), EndoTOFPET-US (GA-FP7/2007-2013-256984), ACTIVE (FP7/ICT-2009-6-270460), and SoftwareCampus program of the German Federal Ministry of Education and Research (BMBF, Förde- rkennzeichen 01IS12057).

References

1. Worldwide cancer key facts 2014, cancer research UK. http://publications. cancerresearchuk.org/downloads/Product/CS_KF_WORLDWIDE.pdf

2. Schulte zu Berge, C., Grunau, A., Mahmud, H., Navab, N.: CAMPVis - a game engine-inspired research framework for medical imaging and visualization. Technical report, Technische Universität München (2014). http://campar.in.tum.de/Main/CAMPVis

3. Delongchamps, N.B., Peyromaure, M., Schull, A., Beuvon, F., Bouazza, N., Flam, T., Zerbib, M., Muradyan, N., Legman, P., Cornud, F.: Prebiopsy magnetic resonance imaging and prostate cancer detection: comparison of random and targeted biopsies. J. Urol. **189**(2), 493–499 (2013)

4. Eiber, M., Maurer, T., Beer, A., Souvatzoglou, M., Holzapfel, K., Ruffani, A., Wester, H., Schwaiger, M.: Detection rate for a novel 68GA-PSMA PET-ligand in patients with biochemical recurrence of prostate cancer using PET/CT and PET/MR imaging. In: Society of Nuclear Medicine Annual Meeting Abstracts, vol. 55, p. 13. Soc. Nuclear Med. (2014)

5. Lasso, A., Heffter, T., Rankin, A., Pinter, C., Ungi, T., Fichtinger, G.: Plus: open-source toolkit for ultrasound-guided intervention systems. IEEE Trans. Biomed. Eng. **61**(10), 2527–2537 (2014)

6. Marks, L., Young, S., Natarajan, S.: MRI-ultrasound fusion for guidance of targeted prostate biopsy. Curr. Opin. Urol. **23**(1), 43 (2013)

7. Mitra, J., Kato, Z., Martí, R., Oliver, A., Lladó, X., Sidibé, D., Ghose, S., Vilanova, J.C., Comet, J., Meriaudeau, F.: A spline-based non-linear diffeomorphism for multimodal prostate registration. Med. Image Anal. **16**(6), 1259–1279 (2012)

8. Schroeder, W.J.: The visualization toolkit users guide: updated for version 4.0. Kitware (1998)

9. Sparks, R., Bloch, B.N., Feleppa, E., Barratt, D., Madabhushi, A.: Fully automated prostate magnetic resonance imaging and transrectal ultrasound fusion via a probabilistic registration metric. In: SPIE Medical Imaging, pp. 86710A–86710A. International Society for Optics and Photonics (2013)

10. Sperling, D.: MRI-ultrasound fusion imaging. In: Bard, R.L., Fütterer, J.J., Sperling, D. (eds.) Image Guided Prostate Cancer Treatments, pp. 115–123. Springer, Heidelberg (2014)

11. Tokuda, J., Fischer, G.S., Papademetris, X., Yaniv, Z., Ibanez, L., Cheng, P., Liu, H., Blevins, J., Arata, J., Golby, A.J., et al.: Openigtlink: an open network protocol for image-guided therapy environment. Int. J. Med. Robot. Comput. Assist. Surg. **5**(4), 423–434 (2009)

12. Turkbey, B., Pinto, P.A., Choyke, P.L.: Imaging techniques for prostate cancer: implications for focal therapy. Nat. Rev. Urol. **6**(4), 191–203 (2009)

13. Umeyama, S.: Least-squares estimation of transformation parameters between two point patterns. IEEE Trans. Pattern Anal. Mach. Intell. **13**(4), 376–380 (1991)

14. Yoo, T.S., Ackerman, M.J., Lorensen, W.E., Schroeder, W., Chalana, V., Aylward, S., Metaxas, D., Whitaker, R.: Engineering and algorithm design for an image processing API: a technical report on ITK-the insight toolkit. Studies in Health Technology and Informatics, pp. 586–592 (2002)

Breast Cancer Detection Using Haralick Features of Images Reconstructed from Ultra Wideband Microwave Scans

Blair D. Fleet[1,2]($\boxtimes$), Jinyao Yan[1,2], David B. Knoester[1,3], Meng Yao[4], John R. Deller Jr.[2], and Erik D. Goodman[1]

[1] BEACON Center, Michigan State University, East Lansing, USA
{fleetbla,yanjinya,dk,goodman}@msu.edu
[2] Department of Electrical and Computer Engineering,
Michigan State University, East Lansing, USA
deller@msu.edu
[3] Department of Computer Science and Software Engineering,
Miami University, Oxford, USA
[4] East China Normal University, Shanghai, People's Republic of China
mengyao@msu.edu

Abstract. Microwave scanning of the breast would provide a technology for cancer detection and screening that is significantly safer than current methods involving radiation. This research focuses on finding the best way for accurate characterization of cancerous signals and normal signals using clinical data collected from a previously developed ultra wideband (UWB) antenna, BRATUMASS (Breast Tumor Microwave Sensor System). BRATUMASS which detects changes in dielectric constants within the breast. The signals collected from the microwave scanning procedure are reconstructed into a single, informative representation of the breast via diffraction tomography. This representation contains the information of the breast's conductivity and the change in dielectric constants. We illustrate the feasibility of using Haralick features to make distinctions among breasts with a malignant tumor present and breasts with no malignancy in data collected from Shanghai Sixth People's Hospital and Shanghai First People's Hospital.

Keywords: Microwave near-field imaging · Breast cancer detection · Haralick features

1 Introduction

Ultra high frequency (UHF) microwaves in the band 300 MHz–3 GHz are of increasing interest for their ability to penetrate through obstacles and perform

B.D. Fleet—This work is supported by the National Science Foundation (NSF) Graduate Research Fellowship under Grant No. DGE-0802267, NSF grant OCI-1122617 and the MSU Beacon Center. Any opinions, conclusions or recommendations expressed are those of the authors and do not necessarily reflect the views of the NSF.

© Springer International Publishing Switzerland 2014
M.G. Linguraru et al. (Eds.): CLIP 2014, LNCS 8680, pp. 9–16, 2014.
DOI: 10.1007/978-3-319-13909-8_2

precise localization and tracking of objects in indoor environments [5]. Moreover, due to their low cost and minimal radiation, UHF band microwaves are being researched for medical imaging [11]. In breast cancer detection, UHF band antennas offer the ability to focus power from the antenna through the breast tissue to localize malignant tumors. Microwave antennas are able to detect very low power signals in the presence of noise and interference, which is important when the target is small and of low-contrast. Microwave breast imaging has the potential to obviate unnecessary biopsies, increase patient comfort, and increase the effectiveness with which breast cancer can be detected.

Detection and classification using microwave breasts imaging has concentrated on simulation studies [2,16], rather than the use of clinical data. Simulated classification studies have used various approaches including support vector machines [4,14], and neural networks [9]. Recently, the feasibility of lesion classification based on contrast-aided UWB breast imaging using simulations was demonstrated [3]. There has been a movement toward conducting more clinical experiments [8], but availability of clinical data is limited.

In this paper, a detection algorithm is developed to detect the differences between cancer subimages (Class 1), and normal subimages within a normal breast which has no evidence of maligancy present (Class 3) based on Haralick's textural features [6]. The uniqueness of this research is the UHF microwave clinical data being used for the detection analysis. The purpose of this detection algorithm is to find the optimal set of features that accurately distinguish between the two classes. Most classification techniques have been performed using mammograms or MRI data, due to the access to a variety of databases [7,10].

2   Background

2.1   Microwave Technology - BRATUMASS

The BRATUMASS developed by Yao [18] is monostatic, meaning one transmitter and one receiver are co-located; the device emits low power on the order of 6.0 mW, and transmits a chirp signal through an impedance matching medium that concentrates the signal for transmission into the breast. The measurements of interest for this system is dielectric constants. The distribution of water content throughout a cancerous breast will differ from that of a normal breast since in areas of cancer, the water content will be more highly concentrated [15]. This will lead to higher dielectric constants in that area. The dielectric constants of a malignant tumor area ($\epsilon \approx 50$) are significantly higher than that of a normal breast area ($\epsilon \approx 10$) at an intermediate frequency of 1.575 GHz [17]. Our research is novel in the fact that (1) the device transmits an intermediate frequency of only 1.575 GHz, (2) that signal and image processing techniques are being applied to clinical data and (3) BRATUMASS offers portability and the safety necessary to allow extensive, longitudinal studies of patients.

2.2 Clinical Data and Data Collection

Clinical data were collected at hospitals in Shanghai under a protocol approved by East China Normal University in accordance with Chinese regulations. In a procedure sanctioned by the Michigan State University IRB, the breast scans and diagnostic data are being used in the U.S. without patient-identifying information. The clinical dataset includes 11 diagnosed cancer patients, with quadrant specific ground truth from the clinician. Figure 1(right) illustrates the transceiver antenna used for data collection, which spans 50 mm. An example of the BRA-TUMASS positioned at the 6 o'clock around the breast boundary is illustrated in Fig. 1(left). As a patient lies on her back, a clinician uses the transceiver to collect data from 16 different positions. At each antenna position, a pulsed microwave signal is sent from the transmitter (A) in the direction of the metal coin slice. The receiver (B) collects information about the changes in dielectric properties from the reflections and scattering of the microwave pulses within the breast, and the clipboard (C) connects (A) and (B). The sent and received signals are passed through a frequency mixer. The output of the mixer is further processed to map the changes in frequency to time delay distributions. These 16 processed signals are used as the signal data to reconstruct a 2D image of a patient's breast.

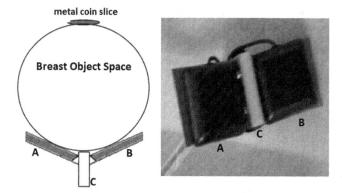

Fig. 1. Overview of BRATUMASS antenna setup, where the transmitter (A), and the receiver (B) are joined together by clipboard (C)

2.3 Haralick Features

Haralick features (HF) have been used to successfully capture textural patterns in images. HF are statistical computations that describe the overall texture of an image using measures such as entropy and sum of variance. Each feature uses information from the gray level co-occurence (GLCO) matrix, which is crucial in computing HF. In this study, the GLCO matrix characterizes the spatial dependence between two neighboring horizontal pixels. In addition to the traditional set of HF, two more features were included, trace median and trace mean, due to the success of using those features for classification of malignant tumors found in mammograms [1]. This results in a total of 15 features.

3   Methods

3.1   Image Reconstruction and Feature Computation

The breast images are reconstructed using diffraction tomography [12,13]. Each data point is represented by a series of intersecting arcs at each antenna position. Each reconstructed image is mapped to a 160px by 160px space. Refer to Fig. 2 for the reconstruction of both breasts referring to patient ID 1, (PID 1). The box in the upper right area indicates the area where the cancer is present in PID 1. HF are calculated on non-overlapping subimages of the reconstructed image. Only those subimages that are not the background or center of the breast are used in this analysis. The background refers to the subimages that represent the air around the breast, and the center subimages are those near the center of the breast that represent the nipple area. Each image is divided into 5px × 5px subimages, over which all 15 features are calculated. The subimage size was chosen after testing a variety of sizes. It was concluded that a tradeoff between subimage size and the amount of retained information is inevitable. If the subimage size is too small, the information in the GLCO will not be retained because the probability of detecting the desired pattern has been limited. If the subimage size is too big, the background effects near the breast boundary will dominate the information in those subimages, even if the tumor is present in that subimage.

3.2   Class Label Generation

The subimage can belong to one of the three different classes. A comparison between (Class 1) 'cancer,' (Class 2) 'normal' and (Class 3) 'normaln' subimages for the sum variance feature is depicted in Fig. 3. It shows the average and standard error of the sum variance (SV) feature for each possible class, across all 11 cancer patients. The sum variance feature is computed using

$$SV = \sum_{i=2}^{2N_g}(i + \sum_{i=2}^{2N_g} p_{x+y}(i) \log p_{x+y}(i))^2 p_{x+y}(i) \tag{1}$$

where N_g is the number of distinct gray levels, $p_{x+y}(i)$ is $\sum_{j=2}^{N_g} \sum_{k=2}^{N_g} p(j,k)$, and $p(j,k)$ corresponds to the probability distribution generated by i, the position entries in the GLCO matrix. In this experiment, the ground truth is quadrant specific, which means the diagnosed cancer location is localized to a quadrant. The key is to detect abnormalities between the normal breast and cancerous breast. Though there are different stages and types of cancer, we are currently

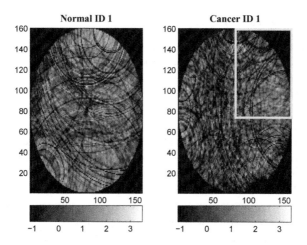

Fig. 2. Reconstructed breast images for PID 1, with normal breast pictured left and breast containing cancer pictured right with a rectangular box indicating the quadrant of the cancer location

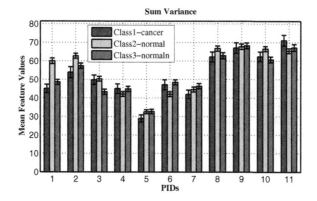

Fig. 3. Mean and standard error of sum variance feature

interested in depicting whether or not there are general differences between breasts with cancer and breasts without any cancer present. Though each breast in its entirety can be labeled as containing 'cancer' or 'normal' subimages in those defined quadrants are labeled 'cancer,' 'normal' or 'normaln' based on the additional quadrant information provided by the clinician. Ultrasound was used to cross check the clinician's diagnosis. Since the only accessible ground truth includes a general area of one quadrant location and tumor size, the difficulty with defining localized ground truth is clearly evident. Creating accurate ground truth is an active area of research.

3.3   Performance Measures

We determined which set of HF best discriminates between 'cancer', and 'normaln' subimages by generating all possible combinations, 2^{15}, of features and selecting that combination for which linear regression resulted in the highest classification performance. The performance is based on two criteria: (1) minimizing the error rate, and maximizing the posterior probability between classes and the (2) Matthew Correlation Coefficient (MCC) [14] score, which serves as a performance measure that normalizes class sizes, and incorporates true positives (TP), and false positives (FP) into the score. This score takes on values between −1 and +1, with +1 indicating perfect prediction. Cost were incorporated by weighting the false positive rate (FPR) by 0.9 and the false negative rate (FNR) by 0.1. As for the MCC score, for every one true cost incurred the final FP was increased by the five to represent a heavier weight. Finally, five-fold cross validation was performed on the two-class dataset, which includes instances of 200 'cancer' subimages, and 748 'normaln' subimages. The best set of features that yielded the highest classification performance by means of classifier performance and MCC score was tracked and recorded.

4   Results

Two examples are provided of the current images used in the HF analysis are shown in Fig. 2. Notice that the distribution of arcs is different between the two breasts within the same patient. In the cancerous breast, there is less uniformity and more scattering than in the normal breast. The lighter pixels indicate stronger changes in dielectric constant. Both the normal and cancer breast contain lighter pixels; however, in the cancerous breast, there is a concentration of lighter pixels surrounded by darker pixels, which is different from other quadrants within the breast. HF are strongly dependent on the images used, which means any slight change in the image reconstruction process can drastically effect the HF numerical measurements, which means extreme care has to be taken with the images selected for analysis. The best feature set can be represented using 0's for exclusion and 1's for inclusion of that feature in the set, which resulted in 010001111111111. This means that four of the features, 'energy,' 'correlation,' 'sum of variances' and 'inverse difference moment' were not used in the feature set. The features included were 'contrast,''sum average,''sum variance,' 'sum entropy,' 'entropy,' 'difference variance,' 'difference entropy,' 'information measures of correlation I,' 'information measures of correlation II,' 'trace mean' and 'trace median.' The inclusion of these features strongly influence the performance measures. The performance measures for the best linear combination of features can be found in Table 1. The accuracy is lower than desired because of the low resolution of ground truth labeling in the subimage domain and the imbalance in class sizes. The more specific and accurate the ground truth, the better the classification that would result. In order to address the issues with class imbalance, the MCC score was used which illustrated more favorable results because of the normalizing capability built inherently in the MCC Score computation.

Table 1. Performance measures of best feature set

Averaged test performance measures	
Classification Accuracy %	71.7
MCC Score	.889

Upon further investigation of features for all 11 patients, it can be seen that for certain patients there are significant differences between classes, as depicted in Fig. 3. For example, for PIDs 1, 2, 6, 8, and 10, the (Class 2) case is significantly different from (Class 1) and (Class 2). This suggests the importance of patient-specific techniques.

5   Conclusions

In this paper, a procedure for selecting discriminating features within clinical data using a HF detection algorithm was developed. The feasibility of using HF to make distinctions between 'cancer', and 'normaln' subimages within a patient was investigated. Due to the differences among patients, it is more beneficial to focus on patient-specific techniques versus across all patient techniques. That is, comparing the two breasts of a given patient to detect possibly cancer-indicating differences may show more promise than comparing each breast singularly with a broad reverence standard. Moving toward a more patient-specific approach is the next area of pursuit.

For future work, extensive studies will be conducted to finalize the most accurate and informative reconstructed images. Most clinicians would doubtless rather have images that clearly indicate the presence of cancer than having to analyze nonintuitive feature representation, so effective image reconstruction is crucial in making procedures straightforward for clinicians. Experimenting with other feature sets and feature extraction techniques, as well as increasing the number and variety of features is another future endeavor. Research is also being done in the signal domain, where classification and detection can be made prior to image reconstruction. Performing detection in the signal domain can inherently reduce the noise introduced in transition from the signal domain to the image domain. Image reconstruction is still needed to serve as a visual aid for clinicians who would rather see an image than a set of microwave signals.

References

1. Aroquiaraj, I.L., Thangavel, K.: Feature extraction analysis using mammogram images: a new approach. J. Comput. Sci. Appl. **3**(1), 33–44 (2011)
2. Bond, E., Li, X., Hagness, S., Van Veen, B.: Microwave imaging via space-time beamforming for early detection of breast cancer. IEEE Trans. Antennas Propag. **51**(8), 1690–1705 (2003)

3. Chen, Y., Craddock, I., Kosmas, P.: Feasibility study of lesion classification via contrast-agent-aided UWB breast imaging. IEEE Trans. Biomed. Eng. **57**(5), 1003–1007 (2010)
4. Conceicao, R., O'Halloran, M., Glavin, M., Jones, E.: Support vector machines for the classification of early-stage breast cancer based on radar target signatures. Prog. Electromagnet. Res. B **23**, 311–327 (2010)
5. Cruz, C., Costa, J., Fernandes, C.: Hybrid UHF/UWB antenna for passive indoor identification and localization systems. IEEE Trans. Antennas Propag. **61**(1), 354–361 (2013)
6. Haralick, R., Shanmugam, K.: Textural features for image classification. IEEE Trans. Syst. Man Cybern. **3**(6), 610–621 (1973)
7. Heath, M., Bowyer, K., Kopans, D., Kegelmeyer Jr., P., Moore, R., Chang, K., Munishkumaran, S.: Current status of the digital database for screening mammography. In: Karssemeijer, N., Thijssen, M., Hendriks, J., van Erning, L. (eds.) Digital Mammography. Computational Imaging and Vision, vol. 13, pp. 457–460. Springer, Heidelberg (1998)
8. Klemm, M., Craddock, I., Leendertz, J., Preece, A., Gibbins, D., Shere, M., Benjamin, R.: Clinical trials of a UWB imaging radar for breast cancer. In: 2010 Proceedings of the Fourth European Conference on Antennas and Propagation (EuCAP), pp. 1–4. IEEE (2010)
9. McGinley, B., O'Halloran, M., Conceicao, R., Morgan, F., Glavin, M., Jones, E.: Spiking neural networks for breast cancer classification using radar target signatures. Prog. Electromagnet. Res. C **17**, 79–94 (2010)
10. Nie, K., Chen, J., Yu, H., Chu, Y., Nalcioglu, O., Su, M.: Quantitative analysis of lesion morphology and texture features for diagnostic prediction in breast MRI. Acad. Radiol. **15**(12), 1513–1525 (2008)
11. Nikolova, N.: Microwave imaging for breast cancer. IEEE Microwave Mag. **12**(7), 78–94 (2011)
12. Slaney, M.: Imaging with diffraction tomography. Ph.D. thesis, Purdue University (1985)
13. Tao, Z., Pan, Q., Yao, M., Li, M.: Reconstructing microwave near-field image based on the discrepancy of radial distribution of dielectric constant. In: Gervasi, O., Taniar, D., Murgante, B., Laganà, A., Mun, Y., Gavrilova, M.L. (eds.) ICCSA 2009, Part I. LNCS, vol. 5592, pp. 717–728. Springer, Heidelberg (2009)
14. Viani, F., Meaney, P., Rocca, P., Azaro, R., Donelli, M., Oliveri, G., Massa, A.: Numerical validation and experimental results of a multi-resolution SVM-based classification procedure for breast imaging. In: 2009 IEEE International Symposium on Antennas and Propagation Society, APSURSI'09, pp. 1–4. IEEE (2009)
15. Wilson, C., Lammertsma, A., McKenzie, C., Sikora, K., Jones, T.: Measurements of blood flow and exchanging water space in breast tumors using positron emission tomography: a rapid and noninvasive dynamic method. Cancer Res. **52**(6), 1592–1597 (1992)
16. Winters, D., Shea, J., Kosmas, P., Van Veen, B., Hagness, S.: Three-dimensional microwave breast imaging: dispersive dielectric properties estimation using patient-specific basis functions. IEEE Trans. Med. Imaging **28**(7), 969–981 (2009)
17. Yao, M., Tao, Z., Han, Z.: The detection data of mammary carcinoma processing method based on the wavelet transformation. In: Wavelet Transforms and Their Recent Applications in Biology and Geoscience. InTech, pp. 77–92 (2012)
18. Yao, M., Tao, Z., Han, Z., Yao, Y., Fleet, B., Goodman, E.D., Wang, H., Deller, J.: Breast tumor microwave sounding, imaging and system actualizing. Adv. Inf. Sci. **1**(1), 1–21 (2013)

Data-Driven Learning to Detect Characteristic Kinetics in Ultrasound Images of Arthritis

Gaia Rizzo[1], Bernd Raffeiner[2,3], Alessandro Coran[2],
Roberto Stramare[2], and Enrico Grisan[1(✉)]

[1] Department of Information Engineering, University of Padova, Padua, Italy
enrico.grisan@dei.unipd.it
[2] Department of Medicine, University of Padova, Padua, Italy
[3] Internal Medicine Clinic, Bolzano General Hospital, Bolzano, Italy

Abstract. Contrast Enhanced Ultrasound (CEUS) is a sensitive imaging technique to assess synovial vascularization and perfusion, allowing a pixel-wise perfusion quantification that can be used to distinguish different forms of disease and help their early detection. However, the high dimensionality of the perfusion parameter space prevents an easy understanding of the underlying pathological changes in the synovia. In order extract relevant clinical information, we present a data-driven method to identify the perfusions patterns characterizing the different types of arthritis, exploiting a sparse representation obtained from a dictionary of basis signals learned from the data.

For each CEUS examination, a first clustering step was performed to reduce data redundancy. Then a sparse dictionary was learnt from the centroids. The perfusion time-curves were represented as a sparse linear combination of the basis signals, estimating the coefficients via a LASSO algorithm. With this representation, we were able to characterize each pathology through a small number of predominant kinetics.

By using sparse representation of CEUS signals and data-driven dictionary learning techniques we were able to differentiate the specific kinetics patterns in different type of arthritis, suggesting the possibility of personalizing the description of each patient's type of arthritis in terms of relative frequency of the detected patterns. Interestingly, we also found that rheumatoid and psoriatic arthritis share some common perfusion behaviors.

Keywords: Contrast enhanced ultrasound · Kinetics analysis · Sparse dictionary learning · Parameter estimation · Rheumatoid arthritis · Psoriatic arthritis

1 Introduction

Arthritis is one of the major causes of disability in industrialized countries: it is estimated that in the US 10 % of the population suffers from limitations attributable to arthritis and 22 % of US adult populations is diagnosed with some arthritis form [1].

Rheumatoid (RA) and psoriatic arthritis (PSO) affect about 1 % of population [2] and are characterized by chronic joint inflammation. RA in particular has the worst outcome and early diagnosis for treatment assessment is crucial [2], but the differential diagnosis is especially difficult at its onset [3].

© Springer International Publishing Switzerland 2014
M.G. Linguraru et al. (Eds.): CLIP 2014, LNCS 8680, pp. 17–24, 2014.
DOI: 10.1007/978-3-319-13909-8_3

It has been shown that a crucial event in the pathogenesis of arthritis (and RA in particular) is the formation of new blood vessels in the synovia, which correlates with the activity and aggressiveness of the rheumatoid pannus [4, 5].

Contrast Enhanced Ultrasound (CEUS) have been recently proven to be a very sensitive imaging technique to assess synovial vascularization and perfusion. In a recent study it has been shown as pixel-based analysis of perfusion kinetics can be used to differentiate forms of arthritis disease (RA and PSO) which did not present significant different clinical values [6]. However, the high dimensionality of the perfusion parameter space describing the contrast kinetics in each subject (together with the possible intra-subject heterogeneity) precludes an easy understanding and interpretation of the underlying pathological changes in the synovium and in the articular tissues. Under the hypothesis that different perfusion kinetics reflect different pathologies and different pathology courses, we aim at providing a more immediate description of the perfusion kinetics identifying the relevant patterns in each patient and for each type of arthritis, with a long-term goal of personalizing the description of each patient's type of arthritis in terms of relative frequency of the relevant detected patterns.

At variance with the pixel-based approach described in [7, 8], in the present work we aim to identify the relevant perfusion kinetics patterns in different arthritis forms (RA, PSO, simil-rheumatoid – simRA, and spondyloarthropathy – SPA) using a dictionary learning technique.

2   Related Works

Data-driven adaptive dictionary and sparse-codes learnt within an optimization framework have been widely used in recent studies and good results have been reported in denoising and compression [9], scene categorization and object recognition [10] on synthetic data and natural images.

Application of sparse dictionary learning approaches on the temporal curves have already been proposed for the study of electromyographic data [11] and dynamic contrast-enhanced magnetic resonance imaging (MRI) [12]. In the first case, the method was applied to one-dimensional motion capture data in order to learn interpretable representations of human motion. In the second work, the method was used to employ tissue segmentation on MRI data, under the assumption that different tissues show different enhancement curves and it was applied on synthetic data as well as on two real datasets (renal dysfunction and juvenile idiopathic arthritis data).

3   Methods

3.1   Data

92 consecutive outclinic patients with finger joints arthritis were recruited, 56 with RA, 19 with PSO, 8 with SPA and 9 with simRA.

The most active joint was chosen for examination for CEUS examination as previously described [13], using a US device (MyLab25, EsaOte) equipped with Contrast tuned Imaging (CnTI, Esaote), and as contrast agent sulfur hexafluoride microbubbles (SonoVue; Bracco International). All patients gave their informed consent to the intravenous administration of the contrast agent and to the participation of the study that was approved by the local ethical committee.

Two rheumatologists performed all the clinical examinations and manually selected the boundaries of the synovial tissue on the gray-scale US images of each patient. Subjects with active synovial inflamed areas consisting in less than 20 pixels were excluded from the analysis (10 subjects), leading to a final dataset of 82 subjects (52 RA, 16 PSO, 5 SPA and 9 simRA).

3.2   CEUS Data Pre-processing

Each examination was composed by a video $I_{CEUS}^{(t)}$ imaging the kinetics of the contrast medium and the B-mode image I_{gs} which allows the analysis of the joint anatomy and of the synovial boundaries, and the drawing of the manual mask I_M. In order to correct for patient movement and to apply the mask to the CEUS data, it was necessary to register the grey-scale I_{gs} image to each frame of the video. Following the approach presented in [8], we exploited the high reflectivity in both modalities of the superficial tissues of the joint and of the bones.

Once each patient's CEUS data were registered on the corresponding synovial mask, the perfusion curves from each pixel within the outlined synovia were extracted. Thus, given the ith pixel ($i = 1, ..., N_j$) in the synovium of the jth patient ($j = 1, ..., M$), the perfusion curve $p_{ij}(t)$ was extracted.

As first step, each subject's perfusion curves were clustered in order to reduce data redundancy and to extract the principal kinetics to initialize the data dictionary. Both clustering methods (partitioning k-means and hierarchical clustering) and principal component analysis were used. The methods were compared in terms of their capacity to detect the different main components in the data to build the dictionary.

3.3   Data-Driven Sparse Dictionary Learning

Sparse representation and dictionary learning techniques were utilized to detect the most frequent and representative kinetics in different forms of pathology: from the components extracted from the clustering of all perfusion curves of each patient's a sparse dictionary D was learned [14], by solving the problem:

$$\begin{cases} \min_{D \in C} \frac{1}{N} \sum_{i=1}^{N} \|p_i - D\alpha_i\| \\ \|\alpha_i\|_1 \leq \lambda \end{cases}$$

where C is the set of all the centroid curves derived from the clustering step, excluding the ones obtained from the subject under analysis. Different size options for the basis signals P in the dictionary (P = 20, 40 and 60 elements) were imposed, in order to evaluate the influence of the increasing sparsity on the representation and perfusion patterns identification.

The dictionary was then applied on the single subject data; the amplitudes α of the dictionary elements for representing each perfusion curve are estimated via a LASSO algorithm with positivity constraint [15]:

$$\begin{cases} \min_{\alpha \in \mathbb{R}^P} \left\| p_{ji} - D\alpha_{ji} \right\|_2^2 \\ \left\| \alpha_{ji} \right\|_1 \leq \lambda \end{cases}$$

In this way, we obtained a sparse spectrum of the amplitudes for each CEUS examination, where α_{ji} is a vector (P × 1) with P coefficients (one for each element of the dictionary) for the pixel i^{th} of the jth subject. A positive coefficient in α_{ji}. indicates that the correspondent basis signal is used to describe the perfusion kinetic of pixel i.

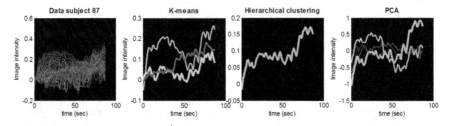

Fig. 1. Comparison of clustering methods performance: example on two representative subjects, where the ability of k-means to extract the relevant pattern is evident.

3.4   Frequency Analysis on the Kinetics Identified by the Dictionary

From the sparse representation of the perfusion curves, it was possible to determine which are the most frequent basis signals used to describe the CEUS data, i.e. which are the most frequent kinetics in the different pathologies.

For each subject j. ($j = 1, ...M$), the relative frequency of each basis signal k ($k = 1,..P$) was calculated as: $freq_k = \frac{1}{N_j} \sum_i^{N_j} \alpha_i$ with N_j number of pixels for the jth subject. Then the basis curves with a frequency higher than a threshold ($freq_k > \vartheta$) were selected (i.e. all the basis kinetics with a non-negative α_{ji} in more than ϑ voxels).

By considering each subject separately we were able to account for the different numerosity of pixels in each examination.

Secondarily, we looked for the more common basis kinetics in each disease type (RA, PSO, SPA and simRA): we counted the number of occurrences of each basis per group and we selected as representative kinetics those at the 10th percentile.

4   Results

In order to assess the performance of the proposed method to characterize a patient perfusion through the learned patterns, we used a leave-one-out validation scheme. At each round of the validation, the data of the patient under study were set aside as test set, while the remaining data were used in the dictionary learning procedure. The learned patterns and the coding of the test data were then recorded.

4.1   Kinetic Reduction Step

Figure 1 reports the comparison of the performance of the methods for the dimensionality reduction. In general hierarchical cluster and PCA identified a limited number of kinetics which were also poorly representative of the pixel time courses (the line thickness is proportional to the number of the pixels in each cluster).

In general hierarchical cluster and PCA identified a limited number of kinetics which were also poorly representative of the pixel time courses. For this reason, the k-means was considered the method of choice and the centroids derived from k-means were used to train the dictionary in the following analysis. An exhaustive search varying the number of cluster from 2 to 10 provided the best trade-off between data representation and complexity reduction when the number was set to 6. Therefore, the set C representing all curves derived from the clustering step is composed by the identified 302 centroids.

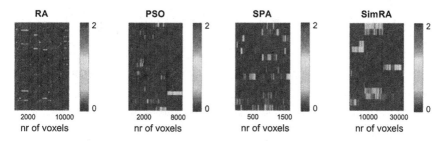

Fig. 2. Amplitude of the mixing coefficients α with a dictionary with P = 20 words, divided per pathology. Black lines indicates different subjects.

4.2   Dictionary Learning Step

The set C is then used to estimate the dictionary D composed by P different patterns. The application of the dictionary and the derivation of the spectrum of the amplitudes showed that, as expected, each subject is characterized by only few predominant patterns (see Fig. 2), as can be noted looking at the small number of coefficients α with non zero values. This held for all the four pathologies considered.

From the spectra of Fig. 2, $freq_k$ was computed for each subject. The threshold ϑ was set to 10 % in order to balance the number of characteristic kinetics for each subject and the ability to distinguish different perfusion behaviors.

The kinetics of the most common words (top 10th percentile) in each arthritis form are reported in Fig. 3. RA and PSO are both characterized by the same most relevant kinetic (a definite slow rising behavior, probably representing a trapping of the contrast agent), namely the basis 102. The second most common kinetic in PSO is still also present in the RA form (even if it is less common). RA is the pathology with the most varied patterns of perfusion kinetics, most of them differing in the value of the delay. SPA and simRA are characterized by a smaller number of kinetics (2 and 3 respectively) but also in this case there is a common perfusion behavior (basis 56).

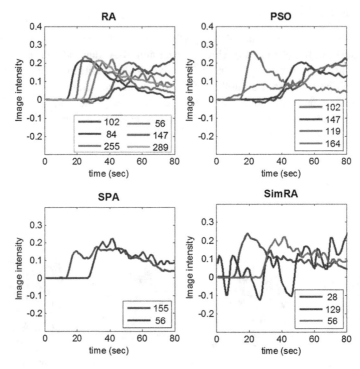

Fig. 3. The most common kinetic per pathology (dictionary P = 20)

The results held when considering dictionaries built with a different number of elements (P = 40 and P = 60 respectively), both in terms of number of characteristic kinetic patterns identified per pathology and in term of common perfusion behaviors in RA and PSO, and SPA and simRA respectively (data not shown).

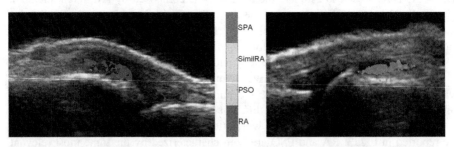

Fig. 4. Representative parametric maps showing the presence and abundance of perfusion patterns linked to different types of arthritis: RA (blue), PSO (cyan), SimilRA (yellow), SPA (red). In the left panel a finger joint of a patient affected by RA, and on the left the finger joint of a PSO patient (Color figure online).

Finally, a parametric map can be obtained showing the presence and prevalence of the different patterns learned as dictionary words (see Fig. 4).

5   Conclusions

We showed that is possible to detect characteristic kinetics in different arthritis forms by using sparse representation and data-driven dictionary learning techniques. We found that, despite the presence of unspecific patterns shared in RA and PSO, and also between SPA and simRA, there are a few characteristic patterns whose presence or absence can provide a strong clue on the type of arthritis.

This unsupervised method could represent an important support in the early differentiation of arthritis forms.

As next steps, the correlation between the dictionary basis elements will be considered, in order to effectively reduce the dictionary redundancy and help the definition of specific perfusion kinetics for each pathology form.

References

1. Hootman, J., Helmick, C.: Projections of US prevalence of arthritis ans associated activity limitations. Arthritis Rheum. **54**, 226–229 (2006)
2. Helmick, C., Felson, D., Lawrence, R., Gabriel, S., Hirsch, R., Kwoh, C., Liang, M., Kremers, H., Mayes, M., Merkel, P., Pillemer, S., Reveille, J., Stone, J.: Estimates of the prevalence of arthritis and other rheumatic conditions in the United States Part I. Arthritis Rheum. **58**(1), 15–25 (2008). A. D. Workgroup
3. Majithia, V., Geraci, S.: Rheumatoid arthritis: diagnosis and management. Am. J. Med. **120** (11), 936–939 (2007)
4. Koch, A.: Angiogenesis as a target in rheumatoid arthritis. Ann. Rheum. Dis. **62**(Suppl 2), 60–67 (2003)
5. Biliavska, T., Stamm, J., Martinez-Avila, T., Huizinga, R., Landewé, G., Steiner, D., Aletaha, J., Smolen, K.: Machold: Application of the 2010 ACR/EULAR classification criteria in patients with very early inflammatory arthritis: analysis of sensitivity, specificity and predictive values in the SAVE study cohort. Ann. Rheum. Dis. **72**, 1335–1341 (2013)
6. Klauser, A., Demharter, J., Marchi, A.D., Sureda, D., Barile, A., Masciocchi, C., Faletti, C., Schirmer, M., Kleffel, T., Bohndorf, K.: Contrast enhanced gray-scale sonography in assessment of joint vascularity in rheumatoid arthritis: results from the IACUS study group. Eur Radiol. **15**(12), 2404–2410 (2005). IACUS study group
7. Grisan, E., Raffeiner, B., Coran, A., Rizzo, G., Ciprian, L., Stramare, R.: Dynamic automated synovial imaging (DASI) for differential diagnosis of rheumatoid arthritis. In: Proceedings of SPIE Medical Imaging (2014)
8. Grisan, E., Raffeiner, B., Coran, A., Rizzo, G., Ciprian, L., Stramare, R.: A comparison of region-based and pixel-based CEUS kinetics parameters in the assessment of arthritis. In: Proceedings of SPIE Medical Imaging (2014)
9. Aharon, M., Elad, M., Bruckstein, A.: K-SVD: An algorithm for designing over-complete dictionaries for sparse representation. IEEE Trans. Sig. Process. **54**(11), 4311–4322 (2006)
10. Mairal, J., Sapiro, G., Elad, M.: Learning multiscale sparse representations for image and video restoration. In: Proceedings of International Conference of Computer Vision, pp. 2272–2279 (2007)

11. Kim, T., Shakhnarovich, G., Urtasun, R.: Sparse coding for learning interpretable spatio-temporal primitives. In: Lafferty, J., Williams, C., Shawe-taylor, J., Zemel, R., Culotta, A. (eds.) Advances in Neural Information Processing Systems, pp. 1117–1125. MIT press, Cambridge (2010)
12. Chiusano, G., Staglianò, A., Basso, C., Verri, A.: DCE-MRI analysis using sparse adaptive representations. In: Suzuki, K., Wang, F., Shen, D., Yan, P. (eds.) MLMI 2011. LNCS, vol. 7009, pp. 67–74. Springer, Heidelberg (2011)
13. Weber, I.M.: Evaluation. In: Weber, I.M. (ed.) Semantic Methods for Execution-level Business Process Modeling. LNBIP, vol. 40, pp. 203–225. Springer, Heidelberg (2009)
14. Mairal, J., Bach, F., Ponce, J., Sapiro, G.: Online learning for matrix factorization and sparse coding. J. Mach. Learn. Res. **11**, 19–60 (2010)
15. Efron, B., Hastie, T., Johnstone, I., Tibshirani, R.: Least angle regression. Ann. Stat. **32**(2), 407–499 (2004)

COSMO - Coupled Shape Model for Radiation Therapy Planning of Head and Neck Cancer

Florian Jung[✉], Sebastian Steger, Oliver Knapp, Matthias Noll,
and Stefan Wesarg

Fraunhofer IGD, Fraunhoferstr. 5, 64283 Darmstadt, Germany
Sebastian.Steger@gmail.com,
{Florian.Jung,Oliver.Knapp,Matthias.Noll,Stefan.Wesarg}@igd.fraunhofer.de

Abstract. Radiation therapy plays a major role in head and neck cancer treatment. Segmentation of organs at risk prior to the radiation therapy helps to prevent the radiation beam from damaging healthy tissue, whereas a concentrated ray can target the cancerous regions. Unfortunately, the manual annotation of all relevant structures in the head and neck area is very time-consuming and existing atlas-based solutions don't provide sufficient segmentation accuracy. Therefore, we propose an coupled shape model (CoSMo) for the segmentation of key structures within the head and neck area. The model's adaptation to a test image is done with respect to the appearance of its items and the trained articulation space. 40 data sets labeled by clinicians containing 22 structures were used to build the CoSMo. Even on very challenging data sets with unnatural postures, which occur far more often than expected, the model adaptation algorithm succeeds. A first evaluation showed an average directed Hausdorff distance of 13.22 mm and an average DICE overlap of 0.62. Furthermore, we review some of the challenges we encountered during the course of building our model from image data, taken from actual radiation therapy planing cases.

Keywords: Coupled shape model · Automatic segmentation · Statistical shape models · Head and neck radiation therapy

1 Introduction

For radiation therapy planning, it is essential to segment vital organs, structures and lymph nodes. Thereby, organs-at-risk can be spared from radiation and the radiation beam can be concentrated on the target areas with cancer cells. Several approaches for automatic delineation of structures in the head and neck area have been made. Teng et al. [10] propose the usage of image registration to accomplish an automatic segmentation. The commonly used approach is an atlas-based model to do the automatic segmentation like done by Han et al. [4], Gorthi et al. [2] and Commowick et al. [1] or a multi-atlas based approach like proposed by Ramus et al. [7]. Atlas-based solutions have proven to be suitable for head and neck segmentation but can result in non-natural deformations when

© Springer International Publishing Switzerland 2014
M.G. Linguraru et al. (Eds.): CLIP 2014, LNCS 8680, pp. 25–32, 2014.
DOI: 10.1007/978-3-319-13909-8_4

image artifacts occur or posture abnormality is present. Therefore, we developed an CoSMo, which is capable of performing an automatic segmentation of the most important structures within the head and neck area in cooperation with two clinical partners. The approach is based on an articulated atlas [8], that is trained from a set of manually labeled training samples. Furthermore, we have combined the initial solution with statistical shape models [6] to represent structures with high shape variation. After the successful delineation of the key structures, the segmentation of tumors can be done using a semi-automatic approach like the one introduced in [9]. Right now, the CoSMo is trained from 40 data sets, which have been annotated by clinicians. We did a left/right mirroring to increase the number data sets to 80, which could be done without much risk because the head and neck area and the involved structures are rather symmetrically. The CoSMo consists of 22 different structures (bones, muscles, glands, ...), which are referenced in Table 1.

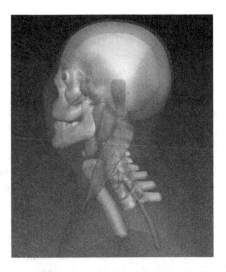

Fig. 1. Visualisation of our CoSMo, trained from labeled data sets, which were acquired for radiation therapy planning.

2 Coupled Shape Model

The basis of our algorithm is an articulated atlas consisting of rigid items for which it already has been proven that it is suitable for delineation of important structures in CT images [8]. In this work, we enhanced the atlas with additional bones, muscles, glands and other structures, which play a crucial role in radiation therapy for the head &neck region, leading to the CoSMo (Fig. 1). The CoSMo consists of two different kinds of model items, which are created from labeled CT image data sets, depending on the type of the structure. They are classified as:

Rigid Model Item Creation: The bones in the head and neck area are represented as rigid model items. For each rigid model item, the segmentation for this specific item is extracted from the training samples. These segmentations are used to calculate a probability image and an average intensity image. Additionally, a relative transform with respect to the center of the whole articulated atlas is stored [8].

Deformable Model Item Creation: The more challenging items, which are items with high shape variation or low contrast, are represented as statistical shape models [5]. For each of these items, a statistical shape model and an appearance model is trained. Analog to rigid model items, a relative transform with respect to the center of the articulated atlas is stored. Additional shape specific parameters are stored, which are needed for later shape adaptation.

The global location and orientation is saved, for every training instance. This transformations of the rigid and deformable model items can be set into relation to the training instance's global location and orientation leading to parameter vector p_j. The parameter vector for the rigid items consists of 7 degrees of freedom, 3 for translation, 3 for rotation and 1 for isotropic scaling. The statistical shape models within the atlas consist of $7 + n$ degrees of freedom, where n is the number of principal components of the statistical shape model (SSM). The concatenation of all parameter vectors p_j leads to a parameter vector x_j for a training instance j and is independent from its global position and orientation. The combination of these vectors leads to a training articulation matrix $X = (x_1, .., x_n)$, where every parameter vector x_j resides in one column. Using a principal component analysis (PCA) on this matrix returns the space of all possible poses and deformations, that is the basis for later model adaptation to an unknown data set. For more details how the articulated atlas is created, see reference: [8].

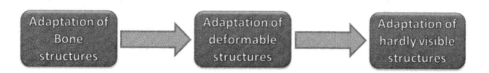

Fig. 2. Overview of the adaptation pipeline.

2.1 Model Adaptation

The adaptation process of the CoSMo is divided into multiple levels, because the adaptation of some model items is more challenging than others (see Fig. 2). Therefore, the adaptation process starts with the items that can be adapted most reliably, namely the bone structures. Once the bone structures are adapted, the next level of the adaptation process is executed. Next, the glands, muscles, trachea and spinalcord are initialized by using the information gathered during the training of the CoSMo, which is used to determine their most likely position. Once again, the adaptation of newly added deformable items is processed. This time, not only the 7 degrees of freedom are considered, but the deformation of the deformable shape models is permitted as well. The energy function for the adaptation consists of the several terms. There is the distance of the whole model within and from the learned feature space, which is used to restrain the model to reasonable poses and deformations. Additionally, there are the energy terms for the deformable model items. These are evaluated using the trained appearance models, returning the likelihood of a valid segmentation. The adaptation now finds the optimal articulation of all items by minimizing the joint energy function.

In the last level of the adaptation process, the remaining model items, which hardly have any visible image features, are initialized and adapted. Constraining the articulation of the atlas to reasonable segmentations of those structures, that hardly have any visible image features. The lymph node levels for example are some of these structures, which even a clinician can hardly see.

2.2   Challenges Integrating the Clinical Segmentations

During the creation of the coupled shape model some challenges arose from the annotated image data we received from our clinical partners. The annotated data originated from actual radiation therapy cases and was not exclusively created for our scenario. While in radiation therapy there is no need for the annotated data to be accurate at voxel level, for less radiation sensitive structures like bones or muscles, in our case the segmentation should delineate the relevant structures as accurate as possible. Since the segmentations are the direct input for the creation of the model items from our coupled shape model, every unprecise segmentation can have negative influence on the created model. One explanation, for the sometimes peculiar shape of single items, may be the fact, that radiologists do the segmentations for each axial slice independently. They focus on what they see in the current slice, without considering the slices they already drew or will draw subsequently. This can result in holes in the segmentation or small spikes (see Fig. 3), which first become visible when the structure is viewed as a 3D representation or when it is inspected in the sagittal or coronal plane.

Furthermore, not only can these inaccurate segmentations lead to unnatural shapes of the involved model items, but it is even more problematic for the appearance model of trained statistical shape models. The worst case scenario would be that the trained appearance model represents a boundary, which is similar to that of another structure and the energy minimization function of the active shape model leads to completely misplaced landmarks in some parts of the model.

3   Evaluation

The results of the coupled shape model were evaluated on 80 data sets using a 2-fold cross validation scheme. Each group of 40 data sets was used to train a

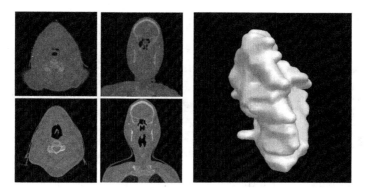

Fig. 3. The images on the left show the differences in segmentation practised by the two different medical schools. It's clearly visible how the segmentations vary in shape and size. The image on the right shows the Mesh representation of a manual parotid gland segmentation by a clinical expert.

coupled shape model and was then evaluated on the 40 data sets of the other group. The used CT scans have an average spacing of 1.0 mm, 1.0 mm, 3.0 mm. The model contains 22 different structures which are segmented all at once during the adaptation process. Table 1 shows the results of our first evaluation. The average DICE overlap for all 22 structures was 0.62 and the average directed Hausdorff distance was 13.22 mm. The whole adaptation process takes approximatly 3–4 minutes for the segmentation of all 22 structures. In addition, the CoSMo was able to adapt to very challenging data sets (see Fig. 4) that, according to a radiologist, are very difficult to be handled correctly by common segmentation tools.

Another challenge arose in the course of the evaluation of the model. The trained statistical shape models of the lymph node levels had an enormous variation in size, shape and even location within the image data (see Fig. 5). After further investigation we were able to figure out, that there is not one clinical practice guideline, every clinic sticks to, but several possibilities how the classification of the lymph node levels can be done. For example, the submental and submandibular lymph nodes are classified as level 1 lymph nodes or they can be subdivided into level 1a and level 1b lymph nodes. There are still ongoing discussions if these subdivisons are clinically meaningful [3]. Although, in a medical sense it may be negligible if the levels are subdivided or not, because combined the segmented area is still the same, from the perspective of training the coupled shape model, this leads to fatal consequences. In our case, 20 data sets from each of these clinical practice guidelines were available. Due to above mentioned divergence between the data sets, we abandoned the option to evaluate the lymph node levels of the CoSMo from the two different clinics, since the results would have been completely insignificant.

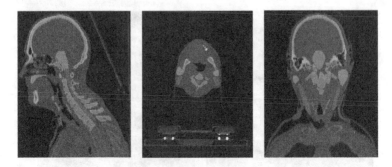

Fig. 4. Example data set of a tracheotomised patient with segmentation result. These patients often suffer from respiratory problems, which require a non-standard posture during image acquisition, causing standard atlas approaches to fail.

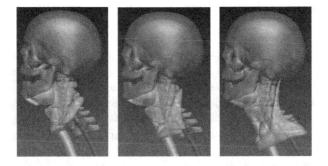

Fig. 5. Variation of the coupled shape model along the first component. The images represent -2, 0 and $2\ \sigma$ standard deviation. It is clearly visible that the variation of the coupled shape model mainly consists of extreme shape variations and translation of the lymph node levels.

4   Discussion and Conclusion

In this paper we presented a new approach for the segmentation of structures important for radiation therapy in the head and neck area. To the best of our knowledge, we are the first to use a hybrid approach combining the clinical approved solutions of an articulated atlas and a statistical shape model. Common atlas-based segmentation algorithms already perform good on some head and neck data sets. Nevertheless, they struggle with images containing noise and imaging artifacts. Moreover, according to a clinician, a non-neglectable number of patients suffer from respiratory problems due to the cancer. For this reason, a wedge pillow is used for the CT image acquisition, leading to a deviant posture, that renders the segmentation impossible for existing atlas-based approaches. But with our method we are able to do the segmentation of key structures and other low contrast structures. Another great benefit of our coupled approach is,

Table 1. Results of the cross evaluation on 80 data sets. The table contains the average and median of the directed Hausdorff distance and the DICE overlap for the 22 structures of the model. Some of the structures, the bones for example, were combined for a more compact representation.

Structure	Ø DHD	Median DHD	Ø DICE	Median DICE
Brainstem	8.16	7.73	0.70	0.71
C1-C7	8.17	6.96	0.68	0.73
Th1 / Th2	12.12	9.37	0.60	0.64
Hyoid	13.60	12.48	0.62	0.23
Larynx	13.38	12.18	0.63	0.46
Mandible	11.81	10.58	0.70	0.72
Parotid Glands (left/right)	17.33	15.84	0.55	0.54
Skull	23.33	18.19	0.85	0.86
SpinalCord	19.48	15.75	0.48	0.50
SternoCleido (left/right)	21.63	20.38	0.37	0.37
Submandibular Gland (left/right)	11.24	11.31	0.45	0.49
Trachea	19.48	18.92	0.53	0.55

that it is really fast. It takes less than 4 min for the segmentation of all involved structures.

Like mentioned earlier, two major difficulties arose while creating the coupled shape model. The first problem is the insufficient segmentation accuracy, which nevertheless seems to be sufficient enough for actual radiation therapy. By remeshing and gaussian smoothing the input data, we were able to diminish minor segmentation inaccuracies, like small holes or spikes. More severe segmentation inaccuracies lead us to the decision to exclude specific segmentations from the model creation step to avoid unnatural model items. As a conclusion, it would be important to explain the radiologists how the algorithm handles the input image data. In comparison to human beings, the machines are not able to realize that some neighbouring voxel belong to a specific region, if the segmentation is not 100 % accurate. Second, the different clinical practice guidelines prevented us from building a model using all available lymphnode level segmentations. After thorough evaluation, it was comprehensible, why the trained model was not suitable for the segmentation of the lymph node levels. Apart from that, it would have to be decided which clinical practice guideline should be used to do the evaluation of the segmentations, as each results in completely different output. In order to overcome this issue, we will build two different models, one for each clinical practice guideline. Consequently making a separate evaluation feasible.

Future work will be to build an atlas from more data sets. This will allow the model to enhance the feature space and cover more possible constellations of the atlas' model items in an unknown medical image. The same applies to the statistical shape models that are part of the atlas. Generally speaking, the results of the adaptation should improve by acquiring further information about the shapes, size and appearance of the used structures. Additionally, more structures which aren't part of the CoSMo shall be included to improve the clinical acceptance of the method. Finally a quantitative analysis has to be done in order to do a comparison with other segmentation algorithms.

References

1. Commowick, O., Grgoire, V., Malandain, G.: Atlas-based delineation of lymph node levels in head and neck computed tomography images. Radiother. Oncol. **87**(2), 281–289 (2008)
2. Gorthi, S., Duay, V., Houhou, N., Cuadra, M., Schick, U., Becker, M., Allal, A., Thiran, J.: Segmentation of head and neck lymph node regions for radiotherapy planning using active contour-based atlas registration. IEEE J. Sel. Top. Sig. Process. **3**(1), 135–147 (2009)
3. Grgoire, V., Ang, K., Budach, W., Grau, C., Hamoir, M., Langendijk, J.A., Lee, A., Le, Q.T., Maingon, P., Nutting, C., OSullivan, B., Porceddu, S.V., Lengele, B.: Delineation of the neck node levels for head and neck tumors: a 2013 update. dahanca, eortc, hknpcsg, ncic ctg, ncri, rtog, trog consensus guidelines. Radiother. Oncol. **110**(1), 172–181 (2014)
4. Han, X., Hoogeman, M.S., Levendag, P.C., Hibbard, L.S., Teguh, D.N., Voet, P., Cowen, A.C., Wolf, T.K.: Atlas-based auto-segmentation of head and neck CT images. In: Metaxas, D., Axel, L., Fichtinger, G., Székely, G. (eds.) MICCAI 2008, Part II. LNCS, vol. 5242, pp. 434–441. Springer, Heidelberg (2008)
5. Heimann, T., Meinzer, H.P., et al.: Statistical shape models for 3d medical image segmentation: a review. Med. Image Analy. **13**(4), 543 (2009)
6. Kirschner, M., Becker, M., Wesarg, S.: 3D active shape model segmentation with nonlinear shape priors. In: Fichtinger, G., Martel, A., Peters, T. (eds.) MICCAI 2011, Part II. LNCS, vol. 6892, pp. 492–499. Springer, Heidelberg (2011)
7. Ramus, L., Malandain, G.: Multi-atlas based segmentation: application to the head and neck region for radiotherapy planning. In: MICCAI Workshop Medical Image Analysis for the Clinic - A Grand Challenge, Beijing, China, Chine (2010)
8. Steger, S., Kirschner, M., Wesarg, S.: Articulated atlas for segmentation of the skeleton from head amp; neck ct datasets. In: 2012 9th IEEE International Symposium on Biomedical Imaging (ISBI), pp. 1256–1259 (2012)
9. Steger, S., Sakas, G.: FIST: fast interactive segmentation of tumors. In: Yoshida, H., Sakas, G., Linguraru, M.G. (eds.) Abdominal Imaging. LNCS, vol. 7029, pp. 125–132. Springer, Heidelberg (2012)
10. Teng, C.C., Shapiro, L., Kalet, I.: Head and neck lymph node region delineation with image registration. Biomed. Eng. Online **9**(1), 1–21 (2010)

Automated Estimation of Aortic Intima-Media Thickness from Fetal Ultrasound

Giacomo Tarroni[1]([✉]), Silvia Visentin[2], Erich Cosmi[2], and Enrico Grisan[1]

[1] Department of Information Engineering, University of Padova, Padova, Italy
giacomo.tarroni@dei.unipd.it
[2] Department of Woman and Child Health, University of Padova, Padova, Italy

Abstract. Intima-media thickness (aIMT) of the abdominal aorta has proven to be an early marker for atherosclerosis and cardiovascular diseases risk assessment in young adults and children. Despite recent studies have highlighted the potential usefulness of its estimation at the fetal stage from ultrasound images, this relies on error-prone and tedious manual tracing. In this study, an automated technique for aIMT estimation from fetal ultrasound images is presented and tested against manual tracing. The proposed technique is based on narrow-band level-set methods applied to the regions surrounding the aortic lumen in order to segment the portions between the blood-intima and media-adventitia interfaces and thus estimate the aIMT. This approach was tested on images acquired from 11 subject at a mean gestational age of 29 weeks. Automatically extracted aIMT values were compared to reference values manually extracted by two interpreters using Pearson's correlation coefficients, Bland-Altman and linear regression analyses. The results indicate that the accuracy of the proposed technique is comparable to that of manual tracing. As a consequence, this approach could be potentially adopted as an alternative to manual analysis for the automated estimation of aIMT.

Keywords: Fetal ultrasound · Aortic segmentation · Intima-media thickness · Intrauterine growth restriction

1 Introduction

According to the Barker's hypothesis, an adverse intrauterine environment results in physiological adaptations of the fetus, which maximize its immediate chances of survival but also increase the risk of diseases occurrence in the adult life [1]. Supporting this hypothesis, several studies have shown that low birth weight, caused either by preterm birth or intrauterine growth restriction (IUGR), is associated with increased rates of cardiovascular diseases (e.g. atherosclerosis) and metabolic disorders (e.g. non-insulin dependent diabetes) in adulthood [2]. It has also been established that infants who were affected by IUGR during the fetal stage have thicker aortic walls, suggesting that adverse prenatal conditions might be associated with structural changes in the main vessels [3,4]. Therefore, the intima-media thickness of the main vessels (e.g. abdominal aorta and carotid arteries) becomes

© Springer International Publishing Switzerland 2014
M.G. Linguraru et al. (Eds.): CLIP 2014, LNCS 8680, pp. 33–40, 2014.
DOI: 10.1007/978-3-319-13909-8_5

an early marker for the quantitative assessment of atherosclerosis risk in children. Recent studies indicate that abdominal aortic intima-media thickness (aIMT) in IUGR fetuses was inversely related to estimated fetal weight, suggesting that the vascular structure alteration could be identified during the fetal stage [5]. As a consequence, the abdominal aIMT from ultrasound (US) images has the potential to become a powerful instrument for the early assessment of risk of atherosclerosis and cardiovascular diseases.

While many methods have been published for the automated measurement of intima-media thickness in the carotid artery (CA-IMT) in adults and children [6], the automated measurement of aIMT from prenatal US images has been rarely addressed [7]. Although the quantification of CA-IMT and that of aIMT appear as similarly-posed tasks, the latter is hampered by several difficulties and limitations when compared to the former. The position of the carotid artery in adults and children does not change over time and is relatively close to the body surface. As a consequence, the US examination of the carotid artery is relatively easy and yields a relatively high spatial resolution. On the contrary, in fetal US the position and orientation of the aorta are largely unpredictable, the vessel lies deep within the maternal womb and its dimensions are smaller compared to those of the carotid artery in the children. Therefore, spatial resolution and SNR are considerably lower, and the correct fetal US examination strongly depends upon the skills of the operator. As of now, aIMT quantification is performed manually on the acquired images. This procedure is tedious, time-consuming and affected by intra- and inter-operator variability, which hinder widespread adoption of this early marker for atherosclerosis risk. In order to overcome these limitations, we developed and tested a novel automated technique for aIMT quantification from fetal US images. The proposed technique aims at segmenting the portions between the blood-intima and media-adventitia interfaces by means of level-set methods and at quantifying the aIMT through shape-based measurements.

2 Methods

The proposed technique allows the automated extraction of aIMT from fetal US images starting from a manual selection of a region-of-interest (ROI) containing the abdominal aorta. First, the aortic lumen is automatically segmented. Narrow-band level-set methods are then applied in the regions above and below the aortic lumen to segment the portions between the blood-intima and media-adventitia interfaces. Finally, the aIMT is estimated on both walls through shape-based measurements.

2.1 Aortic Lumen Segmentation

The user is asked to manually select a ROI containing the abdominal aorta (Fig. 1, left). Starting from this, a simple thresholding based on Otsu's method [8] is applied to the portion of the image contained in the ROI. The result contains a coarse segmentation of the aortic lumen as well as of other potential structures. To identify the former from the latter, area and eccentricity of the best fitting ellipses are extracted from each segmented structure: the lumen is defined as the biggest structure among the four with higher eccentricity. Importantly, the aortic lumen segmentation is only used to initialize the intima-media segmentation step, and thus it does not require a high level of accuracy (Fig. 1, right).

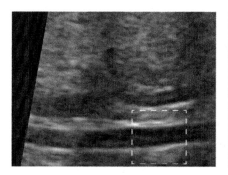 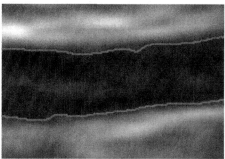

Fig. 1. A fetal US image showing the abdominal aorta (left). The user is asked to manually select a ROI containing the vessel. From this, a coarse segmentation of the lumen is automatically performed (right, red) (Color figure online).

2.2   Intima-Media Segmentation

Abdominal aIMT is defined as the average thickness of the region between the leading edge of the blood-intima interface and the leading edge of the media-adventitia interface on the far wall of the vessel [9]. In the proposed approach, both of these regions - one in the upper portion of the image (defined as upper wall) and the other one in the lower portion (defined as lower wall) - are segmented by means of a single level-set. The initialization of the level-set function is performed starting from the previously obtained coarse segmentation of the aortic lumen: a thresholding process is applied to the two band-like portions of the image which surround the lumen (Fig. 2, left). The thickness of these portions is defined by an arbitrary parameter, which allows to consider only the part of the image where both aortic walls are supposed to be (Fig. 2, left, white). Since both tunica intima and tunica media appear bright at US examinations, the thresholding process allows to perform a first identification of these portions of the aortic walls (Fig. 2, left, orange). The level-set function is initially defined as signed distance function from these portions, and undergoes an evolution in time in order to minimize a specific energy functional in a narrow-band approach [10]. More in particular, the energy functional E to be minimized is written as

$$E(\phi) = \int_{\Omega_x} \delta\big(\phi(x)\big) \int_{\Omega_y} B(x,y)F\big(I(y),\phi(y)\big)dydx \qquad (1)$$

where ϕ is the level-set function, Ω is the image domain, $\delta(\phi)$ is a smoothed version of the Dirac delta, B is the ball mask function which allows to implement the narrow-band approach and F is a generic internal energy measure computed on the image intensity I. B is defined as

$$B(x,y) = \begin{cases} 1, & ||x - y|| < r \\ 0, & \text{otherwise} \end{cases} \tag{2}$$

and allows to evaluate the value of the functional F only in the vicinity of each contour point during evolution. The choice for F adopted in the proposed technique is the *Means Separation Energy* [11], which reads as

$$F = -(u_x - v_x)^2 \tag{3}$$

where u_x and v_x are respectively the inner and outer mean intensity values, with respect to the contour, evaluated inside the mask function B. The evolution is carried out with suitable boundary conditions and is automatically stopped when the change in area of the segmented regions between consecutive iterations becomes negligible.

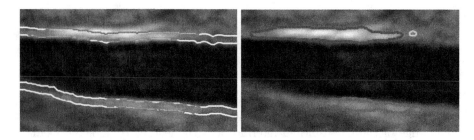

Fig. 2. To initialize the segmentation procedure, two bands of fixed thickness are defined surrounding the previously identified aortic lumen (left, white), and the portions with high intensity within these bands are selected as initial masks for the level-set function (left, orange). After segmentation, one region per aortic wall is selected based on the eccentricity of associated best-fitting ellipses (right, blue region selected for the upper wall, red region selected for the lower wall, yellow region discarded) (Color figure online).

At the end of the level-set evolution, there can be potentially more than one segmented region for each wall (Fig. 2, right). To select only one per wall, ellipses are fitted into each region, and the one with the highest associated eccentricity is taken into account for aIMT estimation (Fig. 2, right, blue and red) (Color figure online).

2.3   Intima-Media Thickness Estimation

Once a single region has been identified for each aortic wall, the aIMT estimation takes place. This is achieved separately for the upper and lower wall by identifying the central line of the region (through a skeletonization process) and by fitting circles in the region itself (with central points taken from each point of the central line): the aIMT value is then estimated computing the mean diameter of the fitting circles (Fig. 3).

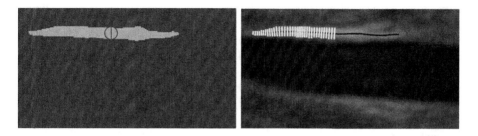

Fig. 3. Estimation of the aIMT of the upper wall from the previously obtained segmented region. The central line of the region is automatically detected (right, black) and for each of its points the best-fitting circle is identified (left, red). The aIMT is finally estimated computing the mean diameter of the circles (Color figure online).

3   Experiments and Results

3.1   Image Acquisition

Image acquisition was performed on eleven subjects undergoing routine US examinations during pregnancy. The study was approved by the local ethical committee (IRB 1826P) and all patients gave written informed consent. Fetal US data was acquired at a mean gestational age of 29 weeks (range 20 to 34 weeks) using a US machine equipped with a 5 MHz linear array transducer (Voluson E8, GE, General Electric Company, Fairfield, CT), with a 70° FOV, image dimension 720×960 px and a variable resolution between 0.05 and 0.1 mm. The localization of the abdominal aorta was performed in a sagittal view of the fetus at the dorsal arterial wall of the most distal 15 mm of the abdominal aorta, sampled below the renal arteries and above the iliac arteries. Gain settings were tuned to optimize image quality. After localization, the vessel was visualized in a maximal longitudinal section (thus containing the vessel diameter) and tilting the transducer to obtain an angle of insonation as close to 0° as possible and always less than 30°.

3.2   Performance Evaluation

To evaluate the performance of the proposed technique, the acquired sequences were manually analyzed by two experienced interpreters (Man1 and Man2). From each of the 11 acquired image sequences, the first interpreter selected 4 frames (for a total of 44 images) based on the visibility of the aortic walls. Both interpreters manually traced the blood-intima and media-adventitia interfaces on the selected images, thus providing aIMT estimation on both the upper and lower wall separately. The proposed technique was then applied to the same images, performing an automated quantification of the aIMT. In order to have more reliable estimates for the aIMT, the obtained measurements (for the automated analysis, Man1 and Man2, separately) were averaged on the 4 frames belonging to each sequence, allowing a patient-based quantification for each of the two walls. Pearson's correlation coefficients, linear regression and Bland-Altman analyses were performed between the aIMT values obtained by Man1 and by Man2 to assess inter-operator variability. Finally, the same analyses were performed between the aIMT values extracted by the automated technique and reference values, defined as the average of the values obtained by Man1 and Man2 (Mean Man), allowing the quantification of the accuracy of the proposed approach.

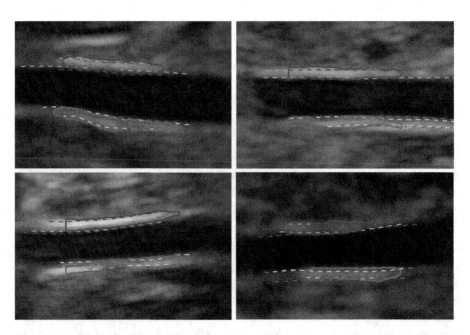

Fig. 4. Comparisons between intima-media regions identified using the proposed automated technique (red and blue, solid lines), by the interpreter Man1 (red and blue, dashed lines) and by interpreter Man2 (cyan and yellow, dashed lines) on images acquired from different subjects (Color figure online).

Time required to perform the automated aIMT estimation for both walls (starting from the user-defined ROI) was around 25 s on a laptop (code written in MATLAB®, no parallelization yet implemented). Figure 4 shows a visual comparison between the results of the automated and manual delineation of the blood-intima and media-adventitia interfaces in images acquired from different subjects: considering that only the thickness of the regions will be taken into account for the aIMT estimation, it is possible to appreciate the accuracy of the proposed automated technique.

Table 1. Results for Bland-Altman analyses. Values are reported in *mm*.

	Auto vs Mean Man	Man1 vs Man2
aIMT	Bias ± Std	Bias ± Std
Upper wall	−0.04 ± 0.06	0.07 ± 0.10
Lower wall	−0.03 ± 0.12	0.10 ± 0.13

The obtained quantitative results for Bland-Altman analyses are reported in Table 1, which shows small biases and narrow limits of agreement (when compared to the mean measured aIMT, which is approximately 0.76 mm for both walls) between the automatically and manually estimated aIMT values on both walls. In comparison, biases and limits of agreement between the values extracted by the two different interpreters are either comparable or worse, indicating that the proposed technique is at least as accurate as manual tracing.

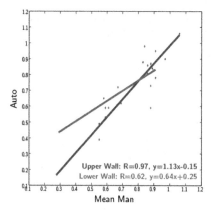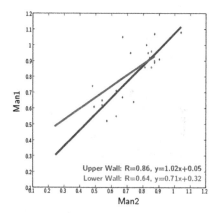

Fig. 5. Results for Pearson's correlation coefficients and linear regression analyses for Auto vs Mean Man (left) and Man1 vs Man2 (right). Blue points and regression lines are relative to the upper wall, while red ones are relative to the lower wall (Color figure online).

These findings are confirmed by the results for Pearson's correlation coefficients and linear regression analyses, reported in Fig. 5: both correlation coefficients and regression lines are similar between automated analysis vs manual analysis and manual analysis performed by Man1 vs manual analysis performed by Man2. Of note, the general agreement between measurements obtained for the upper wall is considerably higher than that for the lower wall, suggesting that the delineation of the blood-intima and media-adventitia interfaces is more difficult in this portion of the image.

4 Conclusion

In this study, an automated technique for the aIMT estimation from fetal US images has been presented and compared to manual tracing to assess its accuracy. The proposed approach is based on the identification of the aortic lumen from a user-defined ROI and on the segmentation of regions between the blood-intima and media-adventitia interfaces by means of level-set methods. The results indicate that the presented technique is as accurate as manual tracing, and could thus be potentially adopted for aIMT estimation in a reliable and robust fashion.

References

1. Barker, D.J.P.: Maternal nutrition, fetal nutrition, and disease in later life. Nutrition **13**, 807–813 (1997)
2. Hemachandra, A.H., Howards, P.P., Furth, S.L., Klebanoff, M.A.: Birth weight, postnatal growth, and risk for high blood pressure at 7 years of age: results from the collaborative perinatal project. Pediatrics **119**, e1264–e1270 (2007)
3. Skilton, M.R., Evans, N., Griffiths, K.A., Harmer, J.A., Celermajer, D.S.: Aortic wall thickness in newborns with intrauterine growth restriction. Lancet **365**, 1484–1486 (2005)
4. Litwin, M., Niemirska, A.: Intima-media thickness measurements in children with cardiovascular risk factors. Pediatr. Nephrol. **24**, 707–719 (2009). (Berlin, Germany)
5. Cosmi, E., Visentin, S., Fanelli, T., Mautone, A.J., Zanardo, V.: Aortic intima media thickness in fetuses and children with intrauterine growth restriction. Obstet. Gynecol. **114**, 1109–1114 (2009)
6. Molinari, F., Zeng, G., Suri, J.S.: A state of the art review on intima-media thickness (IMT) measurement and wall segmentation techniques for carotid ultrasound. Comput. Methods Programs Biomed. **100**(3), 201–221 (2010)
7. Veronese, E., Poletti, E., Cosmi, E., Grisan, E.: Estimation of prenatal aorta intima-media thickness in ultrasound examination. In: van Ginneken, B., Novak, C.L. (eds.) SPIE Medical Imaging, International Society for Optics and Photonics, 83150M, February 2012
8. Otsu, N.: A threshold selection method from gray-level histograms. IEEE Trans. Syst. Man Cybern. **9**(1), 62–66 (1979)
9. Koklu, E., Kurtoglu, S., Akcakus, M., Yikilmaz, A., Coskun, A., Gunes, T.: Intima-media thickness of the abdominal aorta of neonate with different gestational ages. J. Clin. Ultrasound **35**, 491–497 (2007)
10. Lankton, S., Tannenbaum, A.: Localizing region-based active contours. IEEE Trans. Image Process. Pub. IEEE Sign. Process. Soc. **17**(11), 2029–2039 (2008)
11. Yezzi, A., Tsai, A., Willsky, A.: A fully global approach to image segmentation via coupled curve evolution equations. J. Vis. Commun. Image Representation **13**, 195–216 (2002)

Polyp Segmentation Method in Colonoscopy Videos by Means of MSA-DOVA Energy Maps Calculation

Jorge Bernal$^{(\boxtimes)}$, Joan Manel Núñez, F. Javier Sánchez, and Fernando Vilariño

Computer Vision Centre and Computer Science Department, Campus Universitat Autònoma de Barcelona, 08193 Bellaterra, Barcelona, Spain
{jbernal,jmnunez,javier,fernando}@cvc.uab.cat
http://www.cvc.uab.es

Abstract. In this paper we present a novel polyp region segmentation method for colonoscopy videos. Our method uses valley information associated to polyp boundaries in order to provide an initial segmentation. This first segmentation is refined to eliminate boundary discontinuities caused by image artifacts or other elements of the scene. Experimental results over a publicly annotated database show that our method outperforms both general and specific segmentation methods by providing more accurate regions rich in polyp content. We also prove how image preprocessing is needed to improve final polyp region segmentation.

Keywords: Image segmentation · Polyps · Colonoscopy · Valley information · Energy maps

1 Introduction

Colon cancer is nowadays the fourth most common cause of cancer death worldwide and its survival rate depends on the stage it is detected on, hence the necessity of an early colon screening [1]. Colonoscopy is currently the gold standard for colon screening although it has some drawbacks being the most relevant the miss-rate, which has been reported to be as high as 6 % [2].

Combined forces between physicians and computer scientists have been coupled into a field of research referred as intelligent systems [3] which for the case of colonoscopy may be used for assisting in the diagnosis or by providing automatic quality assessment metrics [4]. Another possibility could be the development of follow-up to track a lesion over different explorations over the same patient.

Related with this last potential application, we present in this paper our Segmentation from Depth of Valley Accumulation (DOVA) Energy Maps Calculation (SDEM) algorithm for polyp segmentation in colonoscopy images. We work under the assumption that a faithful segmentation of the polyp region along with a exhaustive description of the polyp region could be potentially used to characterize polyps and will allow a posterior tracking the lesion.

© Springer International Publishing Switzerland 2014
M.G. Linguraru et al. (Eds.): CLIP 2014, LNCS 8680, pp. 41–49, 2014.
DOI: 10.1007/978-3-319-13909-8_6

Our method is built on a previously published model of appearance for polyps, which described polyp boundaries in terms of valley information [5]. This valley information is used to generate energy maps which guide polyp localization methods [6]. Our segmentation method has been developed by considering the way the mentioned energy maps are calculated. We assess the performance of our method by comparing it with general and specific segmentation methods over a publicly annotated database.

After this introduction, we present in Sect. 2 related work on image segmentation, including polyp segmentation methods. We explain our segmentation method in Sect. 3. The experimental setup is introduced in Sect. 4. Experimental results are exposed in Sect. 5. We close this paper with the conclusions and future work in Sect. 6.

2   Related Work

Image segmentation in computer vision is defined as the process in which an image is divided into multiple segments—sets of pixels. Segmentation is performed in order to simplify how an image is represented making it easier to analyze. The partitioning of the image can be based on different features, such as intensity, color or texture, and may not be unique.

Polyp segmentation methods in colonoscopy videos have been mainly applied for CT colonoscopy images [7] or chromoendoscopy [8]. Some simple segmentation methods have also been applied, although they are prone to be affected by noise and other image artifacts—specular highlights, image blurring—[9].

In this paper we will compare the performance of our method against other computer vision methods used in polyp segmentation [5], such as:

- Normalized Cuts (NCuts): The *normalized cuts* method [10] is a graph theoretic approach for solving the perceptual grouping problem in vision in which every set of points lying in the feature space is represented as a weighted, undirected graph. Segmentation is performed by disconnecting edges with small weights.
- Turbo pixels (TurPix): this algorithm [11] starts by computing a dense over segmentation of an image by means of a geometric-flow-based algorithm. This segmentation respects local image boundaries while limiting under segmentation by using a compactness constraint. Regions are refined by using criteria such as size uniformity, connectivity or compactness.
- Watershed with markers (WSM): watershed segmentation [5] considers a grayscale image as a topographic surface and achieves the segmentation by a process of "filling" of catchment basins from local minimums. Providing markers helps the algorithm to define the catchment basins that must be considered in the process of segmentation [12].
- Depth of Valleys (DoV)-based Region Merging Segmentation [5] (DV-RMS): this method assumes polyp boundaries to be described in terms of valley information. The method starts from a first rough segmentation of the input image obtained by means of watershed. The segmented regions are merged using different criteria such as boundary strength and region content.

Our novel Segmentation from Energy Maps—SDEM—algorithm is based on the characterization of polyp boundaries in terms of valley information. SDEM also considers how MSA-DOVA energy maps integrate this valley information o provide an initial segmentation of the polyp.

3   Methodology

We present here our polyp segmentation method preceded by a summary on MSA-DOVA energy maps creation which are used by our algorithm.

3.1   Generation of MSA-DOVA Energy Maps

MSA-DOVA energy maps are based on a model of appearance for polyps which was firstly described in [5]. This model combined information on how colonoscopy frames are acquired with the appearance of polyps in those colonoscopy frames. The model of appearance for polyps describes polyp boundaries by means of valley information. As show in [6], polyps are not the only elements of the endo-luminal scene which convey valley information; image preprocessing should be applied to mitigate the contribution of these other elements such as blood vessels or specular highlights.

The following step in MSA-DOVA energy maps calculation is the obtention of the necessary valley information. Depth of Valleys image (DV) is calculated as a pixel-wise multiplication between the output of a valley detector (V) and the morphological gradient (MG):

$$DV = V(\sigma_d, \sigma_i) \cdot MG; \tag{1}$$

where V stands for the output of a valley detector [5] and MG for the morphological gradient. Morphological gradient is used to add key information about how deep is the valley in the image.

The final step consists of the calculation of MSA-DOVA energy maps, which are based on the assumption that a pixel inside a polyp should be surrounded by valleys in several directions. The calculation of these maps is based on the use of a ring of radial sectors which accumulate for each sector the maximum of DV image that falls within it. MSA-DOVA offered an improvement over sum-based accumulation as presented in [5], using a median operator to calculate the final accumulation value. MSA-DOVA accumulation value is calculated as follows:

$$MaxL(\boldsymbol{x}, \alpha) = \max_{r}\{DV(x + r * (\cos(\alpha), \sin(\alpha)))\}, \quad r \in [R_{min}, R_{max}] \tag{2}$$

$$Acc(\boldsymbol{x}) = \operatorname{Med}_{\alpha}(MaxL(\boldsymbol{x}, \alpha)) \tag{3}$$

where R_{min} and R_{max} correspond respectively to the minimum and maximum radius of the ring of sectors and $\alpha \in [0..2\pi]$. An example of the output of MSA-DOVA energy maps is shown in Fig. 1(b), where we can observe how high energy regions of the accumulation map correspond with the polyp.

3.2   Polyp Segmentation from MSA-DOVA Energy Maps

Our polyp segmentation method—SDEM—uses information from both DV image and how MSA-DOVA energy maps are calculated. Our method requires that maximum of MSA-DOVA maps falls within the polyp and in this case we can obtain a first segmentation of the polyp by joining the position of the pixels that contributed to this maximum—Fig. 1(b) and (c).

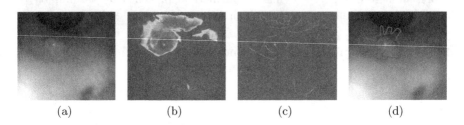

(a)   (b)   (c)   (d)

Fig. 1. Examples of polyp segmentation from the output of an energy map: (a) Original images; (b) MSA-DOVA energy map; (c) DV image, and (d) Initial segmentation obtained by joining the position of the pixels that contributed to the maximum of MSA-DOVA accumulation image. Maximum of MSA-DOVA energy map is marked as a green square (Color figure online).

This first segmentation may present irregularities due to several reasons such as having an incomplete boundary in terms of valley information—see Fig. 1(c)— or presence of spurious valleys from other structures in the scene. These irregularities make positions of maximum of DV image for adjacent sectors being not close one to another—Fig. 2(a).

Our objective is to eliminate the irregularities in order to have a continuous and locally circular boundary—typically associated to polyps—as the contour of the final segmentation. Our method locally explores distances from maxima under each sector to the maximum of accumulation—c^{max}—to detect those positions which are far from the circumference which represents the median of the distances from each maximum to the accumulation center—Fig. 2(b). We use the median distance as a way to correct irregular positions in favor to the most common distance value within a given neighborhood of positions. In this case the use of other options such as mean value are not suitable as the contribution of irregular positions is still taken into account for the calculation. The positions of the pixels source of irregularities are corrected to have similar distances to—$c^m ax$. SDEM consists of the following steps:

1. Calculation of the position of the maximum of MSA-DOVA energy map as
   $c^{max} \in image \mid \forall q \in image, MSA - DOVA(c^{max}) \geq MSA - DOVA(q^{max})$.
2. Definition of a ring of ns radial sectors centred in c^{max}.
3. Calculation of the position of the maximum of DV image under each sector
   S_i of the ring as $p_i^{max} \in S_i \mid \forall k \in S_i, DV(c_i^{max}) \geq DV(q)$, with $i \in [1, ns]$.

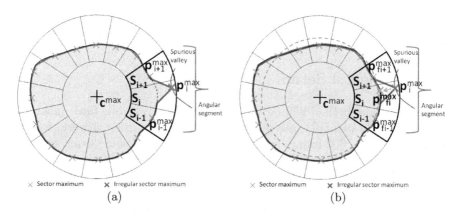

Fig. 2. Graphical explanation of SDEM algorithm. We label maximum under each sector as blue crosses. For the case of the irregularity, we label the original position as a red cross whereas the corrected position is marked as a green cross. A circumference showing the median of distances to center is depicted as discontinuous green line (Color figure online).

4. Conversion of the position of the maximum of DV under each sector p_i^{max} to polar domain $\rho_i^{max} = [r_i^{max}, \theta_i^{max}]$, where r stands for the radial coordinate and θ for the angular coordinate.
5. Definition of an angular segment of size $2ws$ centred on S_i—Fig. 2(a).
6. Calculation of the new radial coordinate by means of the median of the r_j values of the angular segment $r_{fi}^{max} = median(r_j^{max}), j \in [i - ws, i + ws]$.
7. Definition of the new polar coordinates of as $\rho_{fi}^{max} = [r_{fi}^{max}, \theta_i^{max}]$
8. Revert the conversion to cartesian coordinates. The final position of maximum under S_i is referred as p_{fi}^{max}—Fig. 2(b).

SDEM algorithm has only one proper parameter ws which is the size of the angular segment. MSA-DOVA parameters—minimum radii—$radmin$, maximum radii—$radmax$ and ns—are set to the values published in the original paper

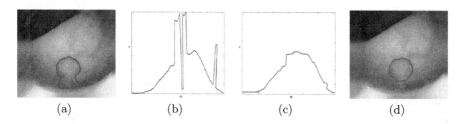

(a)   (b)   (c)   (d)

Fig. 3. Softening of boundaries by median filtering in polar space: (a) Preprocessed image with initial segmentation; (b) Polar representation of the initial segmentation; (c) Polar representation of the segmentation after median correction; (d) Preprocessed image with final segmentation.

($radmin = 25$, $radmax = 135$ and $ns = 180$). To close with the explanation, we present a qualitative example of segmentation refinement in Fig. 3.

4   Experimental Setup

Our segmentation method will be validated on the only public fully annotated database, (CVC-$ColonDB$) introduced in [5]. As in the original work, we will only use a subset of 300 frames from the main database as some sequences were discarded due to bad image quality or presence of fecal content.

AAC, DICE [9] and F_2 score metrics will be used to compare the performance of the different methods. In this case we compare at pixel-level segmentations provided by the output of the different methods with the ground truth. The metrics are defined as follows:

$$AAC = 100 \cdot \frac{TP}{TP + FP} \quad DICE = 100 \cdot \frac{TP}{TP + FN} \quad F_2 = \frac{5AAC \cdot DICE}{4AAC + DICE} \quad (4)$$

where TP, FP and FN stand for the number of True Positive, False Positive and False Negative pixels, respectively.

We compare our method with general segmentation methods—NCuts and TurPix—and valley information-based methods—WSM and DV-RMS—using the proposed metrics. All the methods in the comparison are used with the para-meter configuration described in our previous contribution [5]. We remark that both NCuts and TurPix need to be provided with a number of target regions nr to be extracted. After performing several segmentation tests we selected $nr = 3$ as the most representative result, considering that colonoscopy images present three main regions which are: (1) lumen; (2) polyp; (3) colon wall. For all the methods we used the position of maximum of MSA-DOVA to select the final polyp region. Regarding SDEM, we set $ws = 20$—corresponding to an angular segment of $\pm 40°$—after a training state over 30 images not part of the database.

5   Experimental Results

In order to focus on segmentation, results will be analyzed only for those images in which the polyp localization succeeded. The experiments were performed using as input both the original and the preprocessed image.

We can observe in Table 1 that our proposal outperforms the rest of appro-aches, specially in terms of AAC. Our method provides with regions with a higher amount of polyp content while adding less non-polyp areas. This result is confirmed by F_2-score. Our method provides with a segmentation that covers almost the 70 % of the polyp region—much higher than the other methods—whereas it still keeps a reasonably high performance in terms of DICE. Our proposal also improves the results achieved by our most similar competitor—WSM: segmentation guided by energy maps leads to obtain bigger final regions closer to the actual polyp region.

Table 1. Segmentation results with—160 images—and without image preprocessing—203 images.

Method	Without preprocessing			With preprocessing		
	AAC [%]	DICE [%]	F_2	AAC [%]	DICE [%]	F_2
NCuts	20.29	80.27	0.50	18.02	83.84	0.48
TurPix	19.40	75.56	0.47	14.75	76.30	0.41
WSM	42.89	68.36	0.61	43.68	74.40	0.65
DoV-RMS	56.87	44.93	0.47	54.13	57.46	0.56
SDEM	69.93	69.32	**0.69**	65.07	81.22	**0.77**

Regarding the impact of image preprocessing we can also notice that our method still outperforms the rest of approaches, being our final regions now much richer in terms of polyp content—81.22 % vs. 69.32 %—although slightly smaller. This can be interpreted as our regions being now more inscribed inside the polyp mask, removing more non-polyp content. Image preprocessing also has an impact in the performance of the rest of the methods, being watershed with MSA-DOVA markers the only one in which there is improvement in both precision and recall results.

Finally we present some qualitative results on polyp segmentation in Fig. 4 some qualitative examples of polyp segmentation of several images before and after applying preprocessing operations.

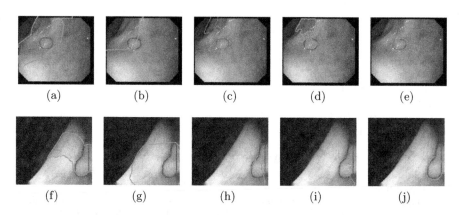

(a)   (b)   (c)   (d)   (e)

(f)   (g)   (h)   (i)   (j)

Fig. 4. Examples of polyp segmentation results: (a–f) Normalized Cuts; (b–g) Turbo Pixels; (c–h) Watershed with MSA-DOVA markers; (d–i) PR and (e–j) Our proposal. Each image shows segmentation output (green) and polyp mask (blue). Top row shows results without image preprocessing, bottom row with image preprocessing operations applied (Color figure online).

6   Conclusions and Future Work

We have presented a novel polyp segmentation method in colonoscopy videos, which is built on a general model of appearance for polyps which describes polyp boundaries using valley information. This information is integrated to generate energy maps linked with polyp presence in the image. Our method explores the way these maps are created to develop a polyp region segmentation algorithm, considering which pixels in the image contributed to the localization of the polyp. Our algorithm is able to improve an initial segmentation by adjusting the shape of the final region discarding some contributions prone to provide irregularity.

The results show that our method outperforms other general and specific segmentation methods in terms of AAC, DICE and F2 measure. Our experiments also confirm the necessity of image preprocessing to improve the final segmentation of the polyp.

Nevertheless our results need to be further improved if our method is to be used to potentially track polyps over different interventions. Future work should consist of addressing the impact of elements of the scene not yet covered such as folds or intestinal content. The algorithm should also be tested on a full sequence rather than on individual frames to test the validity of our hypothesis.

Acknowledgements. This work was supported by a research grant from Universitat Autónoma de Barcelona 471-01-2/2010 and by Spanish projects $TIN2009 - 10435$, $TIN2009 - 13618$ and $TIN2012 - 33116$.

References

1. Tresca, A.: The Stages of Colon and Rectal Cancer. New York Times (About.com), p. 1 (2010)
2. Bressler, B., Paszat, L.F., et al.: Rates of new or missed colorectal cancers after colonoscopy and their risk factors: a population-based analysis. Gastroenterology **132**(1), 96–102 (2007)
3. Bernal, J., Vilariño, F., Sánchez, F.J.: Towards intelligent systems for colonoscopy. In: Miskovitz, P. (ed.) Colonoscopy, vol. 1, pp. 245–270. In-Tech, Rijeka (2011)
4. Oh, J., Hwang, S., et al.: Measuring objective quality of colonoscopy. IEE Trans. Bio-Med. Eng. **56**(9), 2190–2196 (2009)
5. Bernal, J., Sánchez, F.J., Vilariño, F.: Towards automatic polyp detection with a polyp appearance model. Pattern Recogn. **45**, 3166–3182 (2012)
6. Bernal, J., Sánchez, F.J., Vilariño, F.: Impact of image preprocessing methods on polyp localization in colonoscopy frames. In: Proceedings of the 35th IEEE EMBC, Osaka, Japan (July 2013, in press)
7. Wang, H., Li, L.C., et al.: A novel colonic polyp volume segmentation method for computer tomographic colonography. In: SPIE Medical Imaging, pp. 90352W–90352W. International Society for Optics and Photonics (2014)
8. Häfner, M., Uhl, A., Wimmer, G.: A novel shape feature descriptor for the classification of polyps in HD colonoscopy. In: Menze, B., Langs, G., Montillo, A., Kelm, M., Müller, H., Tu, Z. (eds.) MCV 2013. LNCS, vol. 8331, pp. 205–213. Springer, Heidelberg (2014)

9. Riaz, F., Ribeiro, M., Coimbra, M.: Quantitative comparison of segmentation methods for in-body images. In: Proceedings of EMBC 2009, September 2009, pp. 5785–5788 (2009)
10. Shi, J., Malik, J.: Normalized cuts and image segmentation. IEEE Trans. Pattern Anal. Mach. Intell. **22**(8), 888–905 (2002)
11. Levinshtein, A., Stere, A., Kutulakos, K., Fleet, D., Dickinson, S., Siddiqi, K.: Turbopixels: fast superpixels using geometric flows. IEEE Trans. Pattern Anal. Mach. Intell. **31**(12), 2290–2297 (2009)
12. Zhang, X., Jia, F., Luo, S., Liu, G., Hu, Q.: A marker-based watershed method for x-ray image segmentation. Comput. Methods Programs Biomed. **113**, 894–903 (2014)

Generation of Patient-Specific 3D Cardiac Chamber Models for Real-Time Guidance in Cardiac Ablation Procedures

Joyeeta Mitra Mukherjee[1(✉)], Amit Mukherjee[2],
Sunil Mathew[1,3], Dave Krum[1,4], and Jasbir Sra[1,5]

[1] APN Health, LLC, Pewaukee, WI 53072, USA
{joyeeta.mitra, sunil.mathew,
dave.krum, jasbir.sra}@apnhealth.com
[2] Aware, Inc., Bedford, MA 01730, USA
amit.mukherjee@ieee.com
[3] Triassic Solutions Pvt. Ltd., Kazhakootam, India
[4] Aurora Research Institute, Milwaukee, WI, USA
[5] Aurora Cardiovascular Services, Milwaukee, WI, USA

Abstract. Cardiac ablation is currently the standard of care for the treatment of certain types of arrythmias [1]. During this procedure, a cardiac electrophysiologist destroys the substrate needed for initiation or sustainment of the arrhythmia using a cardiac mapping and ablation catheter which is placed in the heart transvenously. Electro-anatomical mapping (EAM) tools have enabled real-time guidance and visualization of the catheter and have additional features which facilitate the procedure, such as, real-time visualization of the chamber surface, ability to tag anatomic landmarks and ablation lesions, catheter display, and activation, voltage (or scar) mapping. Herein, we report on the problem of **surface reconstruction** (SR) from 3D points collected by a novel mapping tool called catheter 3D location system (C3DLS). We highlight the challenges of translating available SR algorithms into a clinical system prototype and discuss our validation strategy. Lastly, we compare our SR results on clinical data to an existing clinical system.

Keywords: Cardiac ablation · Surface reconstruction · Electro-anatomic mapping

1 Introduction

Catheter ablation for the treatment of cardiac arrhythmias, such as atrial fibrillation (AF), often involves the targeting of specific anatomic regions. To perform these and other electrophysiological procedures effectively, the ability to navigate and accurately locate a catheter in the heart is crucial. Several three dimensional (3D) **cardiac mapping** systems are in clinical use [2, 3]. Mapping is the process of selectively moving a catheter throughout a chamber of the heart to determine the mechanism, or cause, of an arrhythmia. Recordings are taken to correlate catheter position with electrical activation at that particular point. Most maps are either activation sequence

© Springer International Publishing Switzerland 2014
M.G. Linguraru et al. (Eds.): CLIP 2014, LNCS 8680, pp. 50–58, 2014.
DOI: 10.1007/978-3-319-13909-8_7

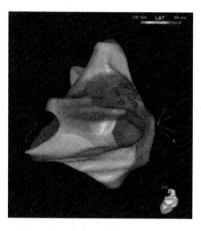

Fig. 1. Example of an electrical activation map of the Right Atrium (RA) created using another existing clinical system. The electrical activation is color coded with orange being the earliest and purple the latest activation. The view is in the left posterior oblique orientation. The red and blue markers depict the location of the ablation lesions (Color figure online).

maps, that display when electrical activation occurs at a particular point as shown in Fig. 1, or voltage maps that delineate normal tissue from less healthy or scar tissue, or simple anatomical models showing chamber geometry.

This work is part of the development of a novel C3DLS tool with intended use on a wide variety of catheters, and has a simplified operation protocol & cost benefits to facilitate wider applicability. A key feature of the tool's software is the ability to generate a surface connecting the points collected during the mapping procedure in real-time. The surface generated must be intuitive and visually appealing, and at least as accurate as the sampling of the chamber allows. The mapping process is semi-random due to the difficulty in precise remote manipulation of the catheter, and may acquire a **very sparse** set of points, based various factors such as, the patient's course of treatment, the need to minimize radiation exposure and the procedure duration. The generation of this surface and clinical validation is the primary focus of this paper.

Surface reconstruction (SR) is the problem of computing a piecewise linear approximation of the unknown surface passing through or close to a given set of points. There are two key approaches to surface reconstruction from 3D points with unknown topology. In one approach better suited to reconstruction from dense noisy datasets, the surface is **approximated** such that not all sample points lie on the surface. In another approach, a smooth surface is **interpolated** from sparse data points, in this case all points are on the surface, noise is assumed to be small or nonexistent. Examples of interpolating surface reconstruction algorithms are Alpha-shapes [4], Crust and its variants [5–7]. These algorithms extract a surface (a set of faces) from the Delaunay [8] or Regular triangulations [7] of points. Examples of approximating algorithms on the other hand are [9–11] where the point samples are used to derive an implicit function in 3D and the reconstructed surface is extracted as an iso-surface of the function. Interpolating algorithms accounting for noise in the data have also been proposed [12]. Some other approaches introduce the notion of flow in surface reconstruction [13–15].

Extensive reviews of many algorithms for surface reconstruction used in computer graphics, industrial design, computational modeling etc. are available in [16]. In the following section we discuss the applicability of some of these algorithms for cardiac mapping.

2   Challenges in Surface Reconstruction for Cardiac Mapping

In order to reconstruct a surface from point data, all SR algorithms make certain assumptions about the data. For example many approximating SR algorithms which determine an implicit function in 3D, rely on the accurate estimation of point normals. Some other algorithms assume sufficient sampling density [7]. In the following list we outline the major challenges in surface reconstruction for the current application:

1. **Point normal** estimation is a non-trivial task for this application as no assumptions can be made about the point sampling density and sample distribution. This is because the current application involves manipulation of a catheter remotely and manual mapping by an interventional cardiologist with restrictions on the length of the procedure to control radiation dose and for patient safety & comfort. Basket catheters are sometimes used to acquire a dense point set in a small amount of time, but the tool design must not assume that a dense point set is always available. This limitation rules out direct application of many implicit function based SR algorithms relying on point normal estimation, and may result in artifactual surfaces when they are used. Figure 2 shows an example surface obtained using an implementation of [9] in the vtk software library [17]. The number of points available to

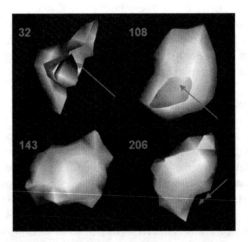

Fig. 2. The surface generated by the vtk implementation of [9] as 32 (top left), 108 (top right), 143(bottom left), 206 (bottom right) points are acquired by the EAM tool. The arrows depict artifacts associated with implicit surface generation and iso-surface extraction. The surface orientations are not matched in all four figures; each is oriented differently to show the artifacts (Color figure online).

build the surface is shown in red. It was observed that the surface topology changed significantly as points were added to the surface (32, 100, 143 and 206 points as shown). Even when there were 200 or more points, the surface was sometimes fragmented (bottom right figure).

2. The **lack of sufficient sampling** also affects the accuracy of the surface generated by algorithms such as Power Crust [7]. Figure 3 shows some example surfaces generated by a vtk implementation of the PowerCrust algorithm [18]. The surface generated by this method has two primary issues: (1) some points are left out of the surface, and (2) the surface is sometimes extrapolated non-intuitively beyond the bounding points. This is mainly the result of the data being too sparse. The electrophysiologist may sample the surface more in detail when the source of arrhythmia is close but most of the chamber is sampled sparsely with total number of points of the order of few hundreds.

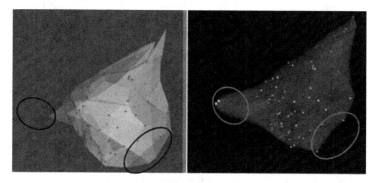

Fig. 3. (Left) The surface obtained from Power Crust algorithm [18] and (Right) the surface generated by an existing clinical EAM system. The same set of points are circled in the two images and illustrate the differences in the surface generated. In the circles on the left of the figures, the points are left out of the surface whereas in the bottom the Power Crust surface extrapolates beyong the bounding points. The orientation of the two surfaces are closely matched but not exactly the same. Slight transparency has been applied to both the rendered images to show points on inside or on another side of the surfaces. No smoothing has been applied to the Power Crust Surface. Topological differences are most prominent near the bounding points.

3. **Non-uniformity** of the point sample distribution causes regular-grid based SR methods to be slower depending upon the resolution of the grid, and computationally more expensive than combinatorial methods which can work directly with the irregularly sampled points. Some algorithms such as the FFT-based reconstruction [19] require binning of the points into a regular grid and have a complexity that is related to the grid-resolution and not the actual data-size.

4. **Visual perception** of the generated surface must comply with what the cardiac electrophysiologist is already acquainted with. To satisfy their visualization need, the surface generation must be real time, start with only a few set of points (about 3–4), connect or pass close to all points, and must be very smooth to enable easy interpretation of the mapped electrical activation displayed with colors on the

surface. The regions with earliest activation times must be clearly demarcated to facilitate localization of the source of arrhythmia.

3 Methods

3.1 Surface Reconstruction

Our surface reconstruction pipeline was designed to handle aforesaid challenges and requirements of this application. The pipeline was developed using vtk library routines for Delaunay triangulation and C++ standard template library for all other mesh-related operations. Figure 4 is a graphical illustration of the primary steps involved.

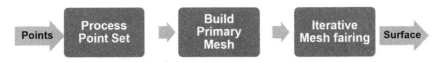

Fig. 4. Illustration of the surface reconstruction pipeline

Process Point Data. The point data are first cleaned to eliminate duplicate points and nearly coincident ones. In the initial stage of mapping when the points are few or nearly coplanar, virtual points were strategically added to generate a stable Delaunay triangulation.

Build Primary Mesh. A piecewise smooth mesh was generated from the points using a combination of two approaches: (1) **A**lpha-shapes [4] and (2) convection algorithm [14]. The complexity of both algorithms is same as the complexity of Delaunay triangulation which did not add significantly to the computational overhead for the dataset sizes encountered. The alpha-shape algorithm generated a surface by selecting a subset of the Delaunay triangulation such that all the tetrahedrons had radius less than alpha. A default value of alpha was used to generate an initial surface. This alpha was determined empirically to be large enough to produce a closed surface. This initial surface may enclose some mapping points, as the optimal alpha for every tetra that would get the mapped points close (<2 mm) to the surface was unknown. Using this initial surface, a more accurate surface with points closer to the surface was derived using geometric convection [14]. The points far from the alpha surface were found first. Starting with the closest off-surface point, the boundary face covering this point was removed and replaced with the three other faces of the tetrahedron which contained this face. Then the distances to all points were recomputed and the process of removing and replacing faces was continued until no more points remained off-surface.

Iterative Mesh Fairing. The last step in surface reconstruction was aimed at making the mesh smooth and visually appealing. This was achieved using an iterative process consisting of subdivision and smoothing. Subdivision methods [21–23] are typically used to produce a dense mesh. A linear subdivision scheme was used wherein each triangle face was divided into two iteratively until all mesh edges were nearly uniform and below a certain threshold. The scalar value at each new point was calculated using the distance-weighted average of its four neighbors. As the subdivision proceeded, the scalar values were repeatedly interpolated from the four neighbors giving a linearly interpolated scalar surface. The smoothing algorithm was based on curvature flow [24]. The mesh fairing process consisted of alternating subdivision and smoothing at three resolution levels starting with the coarsest and ending at the finest level.

3.2 Validation

We used simple phantoms such as a randomly sampled digital sphere and a plastic hexagon phantom to test the surface generation in real-time. As the visual perception of the user is a major factor in the success of this tool, we adopted task-based assessment using human observers. Our gold standard was the map generated by another clinical system currently used by cardiac electrophysiologists. We have thus far assessed our surface reconstruction methodology on **six clinical patient data with the points obtained from the clinical system using three expert observers**, who scored the data on a scale of 1–5 for visual quality and conformity with the gold standard.

4 Results and Discussion

Figure 5 shows the simple phantom surfaces reconstructed from the point samples. The surfaces conform to the original shapes which validates our surface reconstruction pipeline. Scalar values were also correctly mapped to the surface. Figure 6 shows the surface generated by our SR methodology compared to the "gold standard" clinical system. There is good agreement in anatomy and activation times represented by the colors. A small region close to the points with the earliest activation time is demarcated with white color in the map generated by our system. This difference was intentional. The agreement in the colors is better close to the mapped points than in the intermediate regions where colors are interpolated. This is expected by the physician observers who

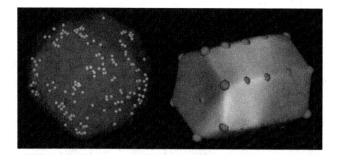

Fig. 5. Rendering of simple shapes reconstructed from irregularly distributed points. (Left) The points were digitally generated using randomly sampling from a geometric sphere. (Right) The points were obtained by mapping a plastic hexagon phantom using C3DLS tool. The colors on the surface depict interpolated scalar values associated with the points (Color figure online).

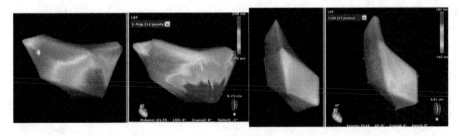

Fig. 6. Local Activation time (LAT) maps for two patient studies, on the left in each pair is the map generated by our system, and the right image in the pair is the map from the gold standard clinical system. (Left pair) Left Atrial Flutter (Right pair) Right Atrial Flutter. The region near the earliest point in our map is demarcated in white.

Table 1. Task-based assessment of six patient datasets by two expert observers. Observers individually scored the visual quality and conformity with gold standard

Patient data	Score 1–5 (5-best): Observer 1		Score 1–5 (5-best): Observer 2		Score 1–5 (5-best): Observer 3	
	Visual quality	Match w gold std.	Visual quality	Match w gold std.	Visual quality	Match w gold std.
1	4	5	5	5	4.5	4.5
2	4	4	4	5	4	4
3	5	4	4	4	4	3.5
4	5	5	3	3	5	4.5
5	4	4	3	3	5	4.5
6	4	3	3	4	4	4
Average	4.33	4.17	3.67	4	4.41	4.17

would usually acquire more points in these interpolated regions to get a more accurate activation time and color if desired. The scoring of similarity by physician observers is not sensitive to such differences; rather more attention is paid to the spatial order of colors which carries information on the direction of conduction of the arrhythmic electrical discharges. The results of the scoring process for the six patient datasets are shown in Table 1. Figure 8 shows the activation time color coded and displayed on the map for two patient datasets. The average score for visual quality and match with gold standard was 4.14 and 4.11 respectively.

5   Future Work

In future work, we will use points derived from the CT data of patients undergoing ablation to reconstruct the surface and determine the accuracy of our methodology. This would also allow us to vary the point density & distribution, and quantify the differences with the actual surface.

References

1. Brockman, R.: Cardiac Ablation Catheters Generic Arrhythmia Indications for Use; Guidance for Industry. FDA Center for Devices and Radiological Health. Cardiac Electrophysiology and Monitoring Branch Division of Cardiovascular and Respiratory Devices Office of Device Evaluation, Rockville, MD (2002)
2. Beukema, W.P., Elvan, A., Sie, H.T., Misier, A.R.R., Wellens, H.J.: Successful radiofrequency ablation in patients with previous atrial fibrillation results in a significant decrease in left atrial size. Circulation **112**(14), 2089–2095 (2005)
3. Fallavollita, P.: Is single-view fluoroscopy sufficient in guiding cardiac ablation procedures. J. Biomed. Imaging **2010**(1), 1:1–1:13 (2010)
4. Edelsbrunner, H., Mücke, E.P.: Three-dimensional alpha shapes. ACM Trans. Graph. **13**(1), 43–72 (1994)
5. Amenta, N., Bern, M., Kamvysselis, M.: A new Voronoi-based surface reconstruction algorithm. In: Proceedings of the 25th Annual Conference on Computer Graphics and Interactive Techniques, July 1998, pp. 415–421. ACM (1998)
6. Amenta, N., Choi, S., Dey, T.K., Leekha, N.: A simple algorithm for homeomorphic surface reconstruction. In: Proceedings of the Sixteenth Annual Symposium on Computational Geometry, May 2000, pp. 213–222. ACM (2000)
7. Amenta, N., Choi, S., Kolluri, R.K.: The power crust. In: Proceedings of the Sixth ACM Symposium on Solid Modeling and Applications, May 2001, pp. 249–266. ACM (2001)
8. Lee, D.T., Schachter, B.J.: Two algorithms for constructing a Delaunay triangulation. Int. J. Comput. Inf. Sci. **9**(3), 219–242 (1980)
9. Hoppe, H., DeRose, T., Duchamp, T., McDonald, J., Stuetzle, W.: Surface reconstruction from unorganized points, vol. 26, no. 2, pp. 71–78. ACM (2002)
10. Curless, B., Levoy, M.: A volumetric method for building complex models from range images. In: Proceedings of the 23rd Annual Conference on Computer Graphics and Interactive Techniques, August 1996, pp. 303–312. ACM (1996)
11. Kazhdan, M., Bolitho, M., Hoppe, H.: Poisson surface reconstruction. In: Proceedings of the Fourth Eurographics Symposium on Geometry Processing, June 2006
12. Dey, T.K., Sun, J.: An adaptive MLS surface for reconstruction with guarantees. In: Symposium on Geometry processing, July 2005, pp. 43–52 (2005)
13. Zhao, H.K., Osher, S., Fedkiw, R.: Fast surface reconstruction using the level set method. In: Proceedings of IEEE Workshop on Variational and Level Set Methods in Computer Vision, 2001, pp. 194–201. IEEE (2001)
14. Chaine, R.: A geometric-based convection approach of 3-D reconstruction (2002)
15. Allegre, R., Chaine, R., Akkouche, S.: Convection-driven dynamic surface reconstruction. In: 2005 International Conference on Shape Modeling and Applications, June 2005, pp. 33–42. IEEE (2005)
16. Chang, W.: Surface reconstruction from points. Department of Computer Science and Engineering, University of California, San Diego (2008)
17. Schroeder, W.J., Martin, K.M., Avila, L.S., Law, C.C.: The VTK User's Guide. Kitware, New York (1998)
18. VTK port of the powercrust algorithm: vtkPowerCrustSurfaceReconstruction. http://www.sq3.org.uk/powercrust/
19. Kazhdan, M.: Reconstruction of solid models from oriented point sets. In: Proceedings of the Third Eurographics Symposium on Geometry Processing, July 2005, p. 73. Eurographics Association (2005)

20. De Berg, M., Van Kreveld, M., Overmars, M., Schwarzkopf, O.C.: Computational geometry, pp. 1–17. Springer, Heidelberg (2000)
21. Catmull, E., Clark, J.: Recursively generated B-spline surfaces on arbitrary topological meshes. Comput.-Aided Des. **10**(6), 350–355 (1978)
22. Doo, D.: A subdivision algorithm for smoothing down irregularly shaped polyhedrons. In: Proceedings on Interactive Techniques in Computer Aided Design, September 1978, vol. 157, p. 165 (1978)
23. Loop, C.: Smooth subdivision surfaces based on triangles (1987)
24. Desbrun, M., Meyer, M., Schröder, P., Barr, A.H.: Implicit fairing of irregular meshes using diffusion and curvature flow. In: Proceedings of the 26th Annual Conference on Computer Graphics and Interactive Techniques, July 1999, pp. 317–324. ACM Press/Addison-Wesley Publishing Co. (1999)

Hierarchical Shape Modeling of the Cochlea and Surrounding Risk Structures for Minimally Invasive Cochlear Implant Surgery

Juan Cerrolaza[1]([✉]), Sergio Vera[2], Alexis Bagué[3], Mario Ceresa[3],
Pablo Migliorelli[2], Marius George Linguraru[1],
and Miguel Ángel González Ballester[3]

[1] Sheikh Zayed Institute for Pediatric Surgical Innovation,
Children's National Health System, Washington, DC, USA
JCerrola@cnmc.org
[2] Alma IT Systems, Barcelona, Spain
[3] Pompeu Fabra University, Barcelona, Spain

Abstract. Knowing the anatomical shape and position of structures surrounding the cochlea is essential in planning minimally invasive cochlear implant surgery. In this work, a Multiobject Hierarchical Statistical Shape Model (MO-SSM) based of wavelet decomposition is created from clinical cone-beam CT datasets of the inner, middle and outer auditory system and surrounding structures. The methodology incorporates an algorithm that automatically segregates structures as the level of detail is increased, leading to a global description of the whole surgical site at the lowest resolution and detailed anatomic models at the highest resolution. This model is the basis for the automatic segmentation of patient data, allowing to quantify the relative position of risk structures in planning the intervention.

Keywords: Statistical shape models · Cochlear implants · Auditory system

1 Introduction

According to the World Health Organization [1], hearing loss or impairment is one of the most common reasons for disability. About one-quarter of men and women over 45 year old suffers from hearing loss of 26 dB and more. Hearing loss is caused by deficits in any of the links of the hearing chain, either inner, middle or outer ear structures. When external hearing aids do not sufficiently mitigate hearing loss caused by hearing deficits in the sensorineural cochlea, which is the auditory organ inside the inner ear, patients could benefit from cochlear implants (CI). Imaging techniques used in clinical routine, such as Cone-beam CT (CBCT), provide enough resolution and context to allow us to capture the structures of interest during the surgical approach to the inner ear, that is the temporal bone, external auditory canal, facial nerve, chorda tympani, ossicles, round window membrane, sigmoid sinus and middle fossa dura (Fig. 1). Knowing the anatomical shape and position of structures surrounding the cochlea is

© Springer International Publishing Switzerland 2014
M.G. Linguraru et al. (Eds.): CLIP 2014, LNCS 8680, pp. 59–67, 2014.
DOI: 10.1007/978-3-319-13909-8_8

needed to plan the best minimally invasive surgical procedure in the mastoid region of the patient (Fig. 1a). In this sense, surgeons can reduce the co-morbidity in patients using direct cochlear access through guided drilling to the inner ear. In this procedure, the most feasible entry path for accurate drill/insertion trajectory is through the facial recess, as shown in Fig. 1b. Safely preserving these structures surrounding the cochlea is of paramount importance for the success of the surgery. For example, damage to the facial nerve would cause temporal or permanent paralysis of half of the face and braching the external auditory canal could cause ear infection [5].

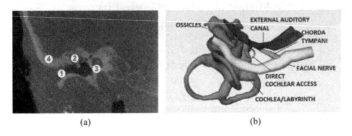

(a)   (b)

Fig. 1. The inner ear: (a) CBCT of the temporal bone. External ear canal (1), ossicles (2), cochlea (3), and temporal bone (4). (b) Example of preoperative planning including direct cochlear access trajectory through the facial recess (Color figure online).

Since its inception in the early 1990 s, point distribution models (PDMs) have proven effective for modeling and analyzing the variability of anatomical structures in medical imaging data, allowing to describe the underlying population statistics from a set of training cases. Based on PDMs, two statistical model of the cochlea were recently proposed by Nobel et al. [10], and Poznyakovskiy et al. [11]. However, none of the surrounding organs from the external and middle ear was included in the models, which limits their utility for preoperative planning. One of the most recent extensions of PDMs has been the development of multiobject statistical shape models, where the characterization of the relations between subparts provide valuable additional information compared to the single-object modeling approach (i.e., ignoring the interaction between adjacent objects). When modeling the cochlea and the surrounding structures, the accurate modeling of the interactions between objects can help to not only adequately deal with undefined intermediate regions but also extract the relevant anatomic relationship between inner structures of potential relevance in planning surgery. However, the classical PDM approach considering a multiobject structure globally (i.e., as a single object) becomes inefficient when a large training set is not available, as is usually the case when working with 3D multiobject structures. This problem is known as the High Dimension Low Sample Size (HDLSS) reduction problem.

For our purpose, good model instance accuracy is essential, due to the narrow space between anatomical structures and anatomic shape differences between individuals. Based on the recent work of Cerrolaza et al. [4, 6], we present a multiresolution hierarchical PDM as an alternative to the classical PDM. This new framework, named generalized multiresolution hierarchical PDM (GMRH-PDM) [6], allows to efficiently characterize the different inter-object relationships, as well as the particular locality of each structure separately. In particular, the model presented here includes the cochlea at the inner ear and three surrounding risk structures: the ear canal at the external ear, the ossicles at the middle ear, and the facial nerve. Finally, the performance of the new model is evaluated in terms of its capability to represent real cases form our database, as well as its potential to generate new valid instances from the underlying population.

2   Materials and Methods

2.1   Dataset and Manual Segmentation

Cone-beam CT (CBCT) images of the temporal bone region, acquired from 7 specimens using ProMax 3D Max System (Planmeca, Finland) were used for this study. The images have an isotropic voxel size of 0.15 mm, sufficient to capture the details of the anatomical structures of interest (Fig. 1). The manual delineation of the structures included in the study is essential for creating a reliable and accurate statistical model. For this purpose, the surrounding structures of the cochlea were segmented using the Otoplan software tool [5]. The ossicles (incus and malleus) were segmented as a single structure, due to their small size, using an intensity-based region growing algorithm after initial seed selection. The external auditory canal (EAC) wall surface was computed from 3 points in the axial view. These points form a plane which moves radially from the ear canal axis. Points were labeled as EAC if their intensity values reached the mastoid bone threshold. For surgical purposes, only the piece of wall located in the facial recess trajectory is segmented. To segment the facial nerve, 10 points were manually selected following its centerline. Finally, the cochlea structure was segmented using the software Seg3D [9]. In particular, a threshold between -300 and $+100HU$ was found useful to separate the cochlea and background/air from the bone. Connected components analysis of the resulting binary mask volume allowed to differentiate the cochlea and labyrinth from the background/air areas of the temporal bone. Once the structures of interest were segmented, the definition of landmarks was performed by means of an iterative cubic B-spline non-rigid registration, defining one of the cases as the initial reference, and using the average shape as reference in subsequent iterations.

2.2   Generalized Multiresolution Hierarchical PDM

The original framework proposed by Cerrolaza et al. [6] integrates multiresolution shape analysis into the classical PDMs. By decomposing the multiobject structure into levels with different degree of detail, it is possible to establish different degrees of association between objects, and thus efficiently model both the statistical inter-object relationship and the particular local variations of each single object. Unlike the original framework proposed in [4], where the capability to model variability in subparts of a single object was limited, as they considered the single objects as the simplest structure to model at the finest resolution levels, the new GMRH-PDM relaxes this condition allowing any possible grouping of landmarks. Next, we present a general overview of the GMRH-PDM. The reader is referred to [4, 6] for a more detailed description of the framework.

Let x be the vector form of a 3D shape defined by $K \in \mathbb{N}$ landmarks. In the general case of a multiobject shape composed of M ($M \in \mathbb{N}$) single-object structures, x_j ($1 \le j \le M$), x is defined by the concatenation of the 3 coordinates of the $K_j \in \mathbb{N}$ landmarks $\left(K = \sum K_j\right)$ that define each object, i.e. $x = (x_1; \dots; x_M)^T$. Using the matrix notation initially proposed by Lounsbery et al. [7], the multiresolution analysis of x can be formulated as : $x^r = A^r x^{r-1}$ and $z^r = B^r x^{r-1}$, where $r \in \mathbb{N}$ indicates the level of resolution (in particular $r = 0$ defines the finest level of resolution, and thus, $x^0 = x$), and A^r and B^r represent the analysis filters. The first equation implements the filtering and downsampling of x^{r-1}, providing a lower resolution version of it (i.e., $K^{r-1} > K^r$, where $K^r \in \mathbb{N}$ represents the number of landmarks at the resolution level r), while z^r captures the lost detail between x^r and x^{r-1}. An optimal selection of these analysis filters guarantees that no information is lost during the process, being possible to reverse the analysis process with the synthesis equation: $x^{r-1} = F^r x^r + G^r z^r$. With this method, it is possible to decompose any multiobject structure into different levels of resolution. At each level of resolution r, we define a particular division of the K^r landmarks into M^r separate clusters, $(S_1^r, \dots, S_{M_r}^r)$, where S_s^r ($s = 1, \dots, M^r$) is formed by the indices of the landmarks contained in this subset, and therefore, $\bigcap_{s=1}^{M_r} S_s^r = \emptyset$ and $\bigcup_{s=1}^{M_r} S_s^r = (1, \dots, M)$. The automatic division of the landmarks into separate clusters at each resolution is based on the agglomerative hierarchical clustering method proposed in [6], where the criterion for choosing the pair of clusters to merge at each step is controlled by the minimum value of the tailored objective function:

$$J(\Omega) = \alpha_1 \int_\Omega \left(\frac{|V_\Omega \times V_i|}{|V_i|} \right)^2 \frac{L_{max}}{|V_i|} di + \alpha_2 \left(1 - \frac{\int_\Omega di}{\int_S di} \right) + \alpha_3 H(\Omega) \tag{1}$$

where α_1, α_2 and α_3 are real values such that $\sum \alpha_i = 1$. $\Omega \subseteq S$ represents a region or subdomain within the set of landmarks S we want to divide into an optimal set of clusters. The first component of (1) takes into account the colinearity between deformation vectors, V_i, and the predominant vector direction V_Ω in Ω. $L_{max} = max_S\{\|V_i\|\}$, and V_Ω is defined as the highest eigenvalue of the matrix $M(\Omega) = \int_\Omega V_i V_i^t di$. The second term in (1) acts as a maximal area constraint, and the third term, $H(\Omega)$, defined as the Hausdorff distance between the objects that compose Ω, promotes the grouping of objects that are spatially close. Finally, the optimal landmark partition is based on the following tailored definition of the Silhouette coefficient for each landmark l_i

$$s_i = \frac{LF\left(min\{J(\Omega_{j+l_i}) - J(\Omega_j)\}\right) - LF\left(J(\Omega_i) - J(\Omega_{i \setminus l_i})\right)}{max\{min\{J(\Omega_{j+l_i}) - J(\Omega_j)\}, LF\left(J(\Omega_i) - J(\Omega_{i \setminus l_i})\right)\}} \tag{2}$$

where $\Omega_{i \setminus l_i}$ represents the cluster Ω_i after removing l_i, and $LF(\cdot)$ is the logistic function. Since a value of s_i close to 1 means that l_i is appropriately clustered in Ω_i, the optimal clustering of S will be the one that maximizes the average s_i. Let now x be the vector form of the auditory system we are modeling, whose multiresolution decomposition $\{x = x^0, x^1, \dots, x^R, z^1, \dots, z^R\}$, is obtained using the analysis equations. Imposing the initial condition that $M^R = 1$ (i.e., a global statistical shape model of the whole set is built at the coarsest resolution in order to guarantee the coherent disposition of the elements), a new landmark subdivision scheme is calculated at resolution $r-1$ for each of the M^r subsets $(S_s^r, s = 1, \ldots, M^r)$ obtained at r. Finally, the statistical model of the shape is created building a different PDM for every S_s^r: $\left\{ \overline{x_s^r}, P_s^r, \lambda_{s,i}^r \right\}$, where $\overline{x_s^r}$ represents the mean shape, P_s^r the set of T eigenvectors, and $\lambda_{s,i}^r$, the corresponding eigenvalues $(i = 1, \ldots, T)$.

One of the main purposes of the statistical shape model of the auditory system we are presenting, is to ensure the legitimacy of the segmentation of the inner ear obtained from a new patient, y (e.g., using Active Shape Models [2]). Suppose that we want to use the new GMRH-PDM to describe a new case, y, i.e., finding the best approximation of y in the subspace of allowed shapes described by the statistical model. Starting from the finest resolution, y^0 is divided into the M^0 subsets previously defined, each of them corrected by the corresponding PDM. This process is repeated at each resolution until $r = R$. In the transition of each resolution, the high frequency component of the new constrained shape, $\widehat{z}^1$, will be used to recover the original resolution at the end of the process using the synthesis equation presented above.

An interesting application of a robust statistical shape model is the possibility of generating new valid instances of the structure under study, providing useful anatomical information of the organs involved, and the interaction between them. In the classical approaches where a single PDM is created this generative process is relatively simple since new instances x can be generated by varying the values of the shape vector, b , within the limits defined by the eigenvalues $(|b_i| \leq \beta\sqrt{\lambda_i}) : x = \overline{x} + P \cdot b$, where generally $\beta \in [1, 3]$. Ho wever, despite the higher potential of GMRH-PDM to generate new instances, the procedure is also more complex. Suppose we are using a fine-to-coarse approach. Thus, at each resolution, r, we should proceed as follows. (i) Generate new instances for each cluster: $x_s^r = \overline{x_s^r} + P_s^r b_s^r$. (ii) Map x_s^r to the shape space defined by $\overline{x^r}$ (i.e., the decomposition of $\overline{x}$ at resolution r). This can be done by simple Procrustes analysis between $\overline{x_s^r}$ and the set of landmarks from $\overline{x^r}$ included in S_s^r. The union of all the mapped clusters defines x^r, i.e., the provisional estimation of the new instance at this resolution. (iii) Obtain z^{r+1} from x^r. (iv) Rebuild the final version of the new instance using the synthesis equation.

2.3 Multiresolution Decomposition of the Auditory System

Even when working with a limited number of organs, the auditory system is a very complex structure, and the typical landmark-based parameterization may be inefficient. In this work, we use an alternative parameterization for some structures, whose geometry can be described more efficiently by means of control points. In particular, the tubular structure of the facial nerve and the three semicircular canals of the cochlea (i.e., the superior, posterior and horizontal canal), are described as a B-spline curve with 17 equidistant control points located in the central axis, using B-spline wavelets to create the multiresolution decomposition. Similarly, the surface described by the auditory canal is parameterized by means of a 4×4 grid of control points. For the ossicles, and the cochlea, the multiresolution domain is defined using the octahedron as the reference mesh, with a 4-to-1 splitting step, and a lifter butterfly scheme for triangular meshes [7], using 258 landmarks at the finest resolution.

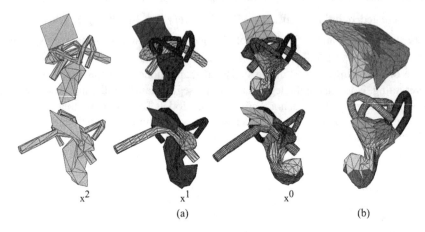

x^2 x^1 x^0

(a)   (b)

Fig. 2. (a) Multiresolution hierarchical configuration of the auditory system obtained via GMRH-PDM. At each level of resolution, each color represents a different cluster of landmarks modeled jointly via PDM. At resolution x^1, the cochlea is in navy, the ossicles in cyan, the facial nerve in yellow, and the auditory canal in dark red. (b) Detail of the clusterization of the ossicles and the cochlea obtained at the finest resolution, (x^0) (Color figure online).

Finally, we create a 3-levels multiresolution statistical shape model of the auditory system ($R = 2$), using 0.8, 0.1 and 0.1 as configuration parameters in (3), i.e., α_1, α_2 and α_3, respectively. These values were defined empirically, based on the general guidelines provided by [6]. The resulting automatic configuration is shown in Fig. 2.

To guarantee overall structural coherence of the elements, all objects are modeled together at the coarsest resolution (x^2). As we move towards finer resolutions, the structure is divided into smaller sets, modeling each anatomical object separately at $r = 1$ (x^1). At $r = 0$, smaller clusters of landmarks are defined on each anatomical object, allowing the model to represent small variances more accurately. At the finest resolution, it is possible to observe an anatomical correspondence between the clusters obtained and the different anatomical subregions of the ossicles: malleus (light blue), handle of malleus (red), long process of incus (light orange); and the cochlea: semi-circular canals (yellow, green and dark blue), cochlear duct (dark blue), tympanic duct (light green) (see Fig. 1b).

3 Results and Discussion

The ability of the new statistical shape model to represent new instances of the underlying population is evaluated in terms of the average landmark-to-landmark distance (L2L), the landmark-to-surface distance (L2S), and the Dice coefficient (DC), using leave-one-out cross-validation. Table 1 shows the results obtained for each one of the organs included in this study. The average L2L error for each landmark is shown in Fig. 3(a). As it can be observed in Table 1, a better accuracy is obtained for the cochlea (including the cochlear canals) and the ossicles, with an error below 0.45 mm (L2L and L2S), and a DC greater than 0.78. On the other hand, the facial nerve and the auditory canal have an average L2S error of 1.16 mm and 1.17 mm, respectively. In the context of surgical planning of cochlear implants, the narrow space between risk structures results in a need of systems with high accuracy, preferably below 1 mm [8]. The promising results obtained for the cochlea and ossicles shows the potential of the statistical model presented here for such demanding applications, though further work is needed in order to improve the accuracy in the remaining structures, the facial nerve and the auditory canal. Finally, as Sect. 2.2 indicates, the new statistical model generated via GMRH-PDM is able to generate a wide variety of new valid instances thanks to the multiresolution shape decomposition and the creation of small clusters of landmarks, of great utility in the anatomical study of the auditory system, and the spatial relationship between the organs. Figure 3(b) shows a set of new cases randomly generated by the model ($\beta = 2$). These instances were evaluated by an expert radiologist who verified satisfactorily the anatomical validity of the structures.

Table 1. Accuracy Evaluation of the statistical shape model. Landmark-to-landmark (L2L) distance, landmark-to-surface (L2S) distance, and Dice coefficient (DC) for the seven objects considered here: cochlea, superior canal (Sup. C.), posterior canal (Pos. C), horizontal canal (Hor. C), ossicles (Oss.), facial nerve (Facial N.) and auditory canal (Audit. C.). The Audit. C is represented by an open surface, so no DC can be calculated.

	Cochlea	Sup. C.	Pos. C.	Hor. C	Oss.	Facial. N.	Audit. C.
L2L (mm)	0.32 ± 0.06	0.64 ± 0.12	0.60 ± 0.12	0.75 ± 0.24	0.45 ± 0.11	1.15 ± 0.19	1.30 ± 0.41
L2S (mm)	0.25 ± 0.04	0.64 ± 0.11	0.55 ± 0.12	0.72 ± 0.20	0.38 ± 0.10	1.16 ± 0.31	1.17 ± 0.35
DC	0.89 ± 0.02	0.75 ± 0.03	0.76 ± 0.07	0.70 ± 0.14	0.78 ± 0.04	0.60 ± 0.10	–

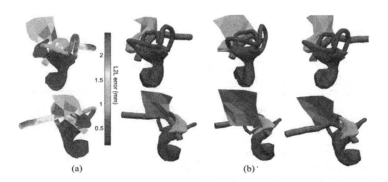

(a)   (b)

Fig. 3. Performance characterization of the statistical shape model of the auditory system. (a) Average L2L error for each landmark. (b) Example of the ability of the GMRH-PDM to generate new valid instances of the auditory system ($\beta = 2$).

4 Conclusion

Cochlear implantation requires accurate planning of the surgical intervention in order to reduce co-morbidity in patients when using direct cochlear access through guided drilling to the inner ear. Therefore, knowledge of the anatomical shape and location of the surrounding structures is essential. Based on the new GMRH-PDM framework, this paper presents a new statistical shape model of the auditory system consisting of the cochlea, the ossicles, the facial nerve, and the auditory canal. This new approach allows to describe efficiently the variability of the structures under study at different levels of resolution, guaranteeing that only valid instances are generated. In this paper we show the potential of the new statistical model of the auditory system to model new instances (average L2S error = 0.70 ± 0.36 mm), even when a limited number of training cases is available. We plan to continue exploiting the capacity of the multiresolution hierarchical modeling to create a more complete anatomical model of the auditory system, including other important organs like the temporal bone, and the chorda tympani.

Acknowledgment. This project was supported by a philanthropic gift from the Government of Abu Dhabi to Children's National Health System, and by the European Union FP7 project HEAR-EU (grant agreement 304857).

References

1. The global burden of disease. World Health Organization (2004)
2. Cootes, T.F., et al.: Active shape modelstheir training and application. Comput. Vis. Image Underst. **61**(1), 38–59 (1995)
3. Duta, N., Sonka, M.: Segmentation and interpretation of MR brain images an improved active shape model. IEEE Trans. Med. Imag. **17**(6), 1049–1062 (1998)
4. Cerrolaza, J.J., et al.: Hierarchical statistical shape models of multiobject anatomical structures: application to brain MRI. IEEE Trans. Med. Imaging **31**(3), 71–724 (2012)
5. Gerber, N., et al.: Surgical planning tool for robotically assisted hearing aid implantation. Int. J. Comp. Ass. Rad. Sur. **9**(1), 11–20 (2013, 2014)
6. Cerrolaza, J.J., Villanueva, A., Reyes, M., Cabeza, R., González Ballester, M.A., Linguraru, M.G.: Generalized multiresolution hierarchical shape models via automatic landmark clusterization. In: Golland, P., Hata, N., Barillot, C., Hornegger, J., Howe, R. (eds.) MICCAI 2014, Part III. LNCS, vol. 8675, pp. 1–8. Springer, Heidelberg (2014)
7. Dyn, N., et al.: A butterfly subdivision scheme for surface interpolation with tension control. ACM Trans. Graph. **9**(2), 160–169 (1990)
8. Noble, J.H., et al.: Automatic determination of optimal linear drilling trajectories for cochlear access accounting for drill positioning error. Int. J. Med. Robot. **6**(3), 281–290 (2011)
9. Center for Integrative Biomedical Computing (CIBC), University of Utah Scientific Computing and Imaging (SCI) Institute. Seg3D: Volumetric Image Segmentation and Visualization (2013). http://www.seg3d.org

10. Noble, J.H., Gifford, R.H., Labadie, R.F., Dawant, B.M.: Statistical shape model segmentation and frequency mapping of cochlear implant stimulation targets in CT. In: Ayache, N., Delingette, H., Golland, P., Mori, K. (eds.) MICCAI 2012, Part II. LNCS, vol. 7511, pp. 421–428. Springer, Heidelberg (2012)
11. Poznyakovskiy, A.A., et al.: Statistical shape modeling of human cochlea: Alignment and principal component analysis. In: Proceedings of the SPIE 8670 Medical Imaging (2013)

Noninvasive Electrocardiographic Imaging of Cardiac Arrhythmias: Enhance the Diagnosis of Bundle Branch Block

Liansheng Wang[1,2(✉)], Yiping Chen[1,3], Huangjing Lin[1], and Dong Ni[2]

[1] Department of Computer Science, School of Information Science and Engineering,
Xiamen University, Xiamen, China
lswang@xmu.edu.cn
[2] Guangdong Key Laboratory for Biomedical Measurements and Ultrasound
Imaging, Shenzhen 518060, China
[3] College of Electronic Science and Engineering,
National University of Defense Technology, Changsha, China

Abstract. Bundle Branch Block (BBB) is a heart disease which is usually diagnosed by the analysis of the ECG morphology and the duration of its QRS complex. Although body surface potential mapping (BSPM) provides more information than 12-lead ECG and is noninvasive, it is still not a visually direct method like in 3D heart model. In this paper we aim to propose a system in which the 3D transmembrane potential is estimated and visualized in the 3D heart model to improve the diagnosis of BBB. Using patient CT and BSPM data, the system is able to reconstruct details of the complete electrical activity of BBB on the 3D heart model. With the quantitative analysis proposed, BBB patterns can be more easily distinguished in 3D model than by visual inspection of the standard ECG and BSPM, therefore enhancing BBB diagnosis for the physicians.

Keywords: CT images · Bundle branch block · Noninvasive imaging · 3D

1 Introduction

Bundle branch block (BBB) is a heart disease. It is caused when one of the branches, or of the fascicles, of the bundle cannot normally transmit the electrical impulses. These electrical impulses will cause ventricular contraction. Therefore, in order to work normally, these impulses have to be transmitted by another path which eventually cause both ventricles do not contract simultaneously. In routine treatment, diagnosis of BBB is based on recognization of the ECG signal pattern and on the duration of the QRS complex [1].

Although the 12-lead ECG is the most common used technique in cardiology, several studies have been conducted in order to determine if the use of more leads would provide more information [2]. In the BSPM system, there are usually 30 or more electrodes using for collecting the potential information on the torso

© Springer International Publishing Switzerland 2014
M.G. Linguraru et al. (Eds.): CLIP 2014, LNCS 8680, pp. 68–75, 2014.
DOI: 10.1007/978-3-319-13909-8_9

surface [3]. These body surface potentials collected reflect the activity of heart. Since BSPM have more electrodes than ECG, BSPM thus provide more information about heart [4].

By employing BSPM, the basic information of heart is easily to be reconstructed. It thus provides the spatiotemporal functional information of the underlying cardiac electrical activity [5]. Hence, it is possible to observe the activation pattern for a specific pacing site and this can be more useful than ECG in the diagnosis of heart diseases, such as BBB. While great efforts have been paid to build up BSPM database for diagnosis of heart disease [6], BSPM is not able to reflect local detailed information of the electrical activity in the 3D heart model, since each electrode on the torso actually only remotely measures a smoothed integration of the entire cardiac activity [5].

Although lots of previous works have been done on using BSPM system to enhance the diagnosis of BBB [7], there has no actual effort to enhance its diagnosis more directly using BSPM in the 3D heart model. Previous studies have no clinical usefulness because they only reported quantitatively different map patterns in potential maps. Donis et al. studied 64-lead BSPM recordings to improve the diagnosis of BBB compared with the 12 standard leads of ECG. But the results are simple and not visually realistic like in 3D myocardium for physicians [8]. Auricchio et al. used catheter electrical recording to map the electrical events on the hear model. Although their method gave a higher sensitivity to rapidly changing events in the hear model and is useful for identifying and locating specific locations, their method is invasive [9].

In this study, the BSPM of patients with BBB were measured and used to reconstruct the epicardial potential to analyze whether other subjects have BBB or not in 3D heart model. With BSPM data collected from patients with BBB, 3D dynamic geometry heart model is non-invasively built [6]. The evaluation of diagnosis of BBB is compared to previous studies and physicians' interpretation of the infarct BBB. If the similar activation patterns can be found, corresponding epicardial potential maps in 3D heart model will be generated and saved. Then we can automatically classify patients using the representative maps, in which these patients have the similarity of activity pattern in 3D. Thus the proposed system helps the physicians to improve the diagnosis of BBB.

2   Method

The whole overview of our system is illustrated in Fig. 1. In the presented study, we aim to estimate the epicardial potential distribution on the 3D myocardium from noninvasive measured BSPM, in which the anatomic data for building heart and torso model obtained from computed tomography (CT) image sequences and a priori information of cardiac electrophysiology. The epicardial potential distribution is reconstructed using BSPM with a patient specific heart-torso geometry model.

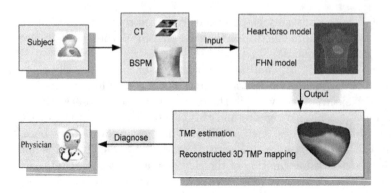

Fig. 1. Overview of the whole proposed system.

2.1   Forward and Inverse Model

Assuming the human torso is homogeneous and isotropic, boundary element method (BEM) [10] is applied to discretize the torso and the epicardial surfaces to derive a relationship between torso potentials and epicardial potentials:

$$\Phi_T = \mathbf{A}\Phi_E \tag{1}$$

where m-dimensional vector Φ_T is the potentials on the torso surface and n-dimensional vector Φ_E is the potentials on the epicardial surface, $(m * n)$ $(n < m)$ matrix A is a transfer matrix. The transfer matrix $\mathbf{A}$ depends entirely on the boundary integrands of Laplace's equation, which can be estimated analytically using BEM from a solution of forward problem. The epicardial surface (490 nodes and 976 triangles) is obtained from CT scans in human studies, while the torso surface (coordinates) (771 nodes and 1254 triangles) is from the position of electrodes on the torso.

Based on the forward solution, we use our previous proposed method [11] to estimate the epicardial potentials. The method is a L1-norm based inverse solution which can reduce the computational complexity and make rapid convergence possible.

2.2   Epicardial Potential Estimation and Imaging

The architecture of this noninvasive TMP imaging system is illustrated in Fig. 1. Priori physiological knowledge and patient data were combined together, in which their respective uncertainties are considered. Physiologically geometry heart model and torso model were built from MRI image sequences. FHN model is employed for the system to generated potential propagation and to compared with the results of inverse problem. Then the epicardial potential is reconstructed using the techniques of ECG inverse problem. And the activation maps will be calculated for evaluation [12].

3   Experiments and Results

3.1   Data

The ECG recordings were collected using a BSPM system. BSPM system used in this study is a commercial 73-lead recording system for biopotential measurements (called Active One). The quantization rate was 1 microvolt per bit and the sampling rate used in the BSPM system was 2048 Hz. Electrodes were distributed non-uniformly when capture the BSPM, where 19 electrodes were on the back and 54 on the front. Therefore, we got higher electrode density at position of the heart (see Fig. 2(a)).

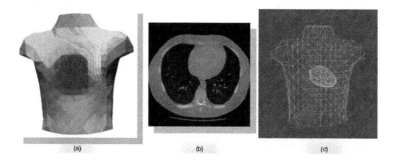

Fig. 2. Input data (a) BSPM; (b) CT data; (c) heart-torso model.

In order to improve the effectivity of signal of BSPM, the BSPM were preprocessed using filters. Preprocessing of patient BSP data is necessary to coordinate the real data with the physiological system. We select QRS intervals out of the complete BSPM which will be further interpolated as input for the system. Table 1 shows the mean value of QRS duration using this preprocessing.

Table 1. Mean value of QRS duration (in ms (milliseconds)) after the preprocessing for each category of patients.

Category	12-lead ECG	74-lead BSPM
Healthy (n = 9)	114.0 ± 5.1	121.1 ± 12.4
All BBB (n = 18)	173.1 ± 30	185.5 ± 26.7
LBBB (n = 13)	180.4 ± 22.1	193.2 ± 21.5
RBBB (n = 5)	150.0 ± 16.5	171.1 ± 15.1

The geometry heart and torso model were reconstructed using CT image sequences of a patient (see Fig. 2(b)). The torso surface and epicardial surface were divided into 490 and 976 nodes, and 771, 1254 triangles, respectively.

The heart surface mesh were achieved manually and there are 2500 points in the mesh. We also used a mathematical fibrous model [2] to simulate the anisotropic myocardial conductive. The torso is assumed to have an isotropic and homogeneous conduction, which is described by triangulated body surface with 347 apexes and built by matching a reference torso model with patient's CT data sequences [13]. Figure 2(c) illustrates the heart-torso model.

3.2   Population Under Study

In order to comprehensively evaluate the system, we collected data from both normal subjects and patients with BBB. For the ECG BSPM recordings, the time for capturing is one minute. In all these data, there 18 data were collected from patients with BBB and 9 data from healthy persons. Diagnosis of subjects under this study is listed in Table 2.

Table 2. The number of subjects in our experiments.

Diagnosis	Number of patients
Total	27
Healthy	9
Complete left BBB (LBBB)	13
Complete right BBB (RBBB) & anterior hemiblock (RBBB_AH)	5

3.3   Results and Discussion

Epicardial potential mapping showed that from the pacing site of earliest LV activation, activation wavefronts spread naturally with high fidelity or not. For some patients, the activation wavefronts could not spread directly to the lateral wall from the anterior region. Instead, this wavefront spreads inferiorly around the apex and across the inferior wall, then reached the lateral or posterolateral regions. LV activation finally reach the basal region near the mitral valve annulus. This pattern of activation was observed in some patients's data. The accuracy of TMP estimates is also validated by the closeness between estimates-generated TMP and the input data (see Figs. 4 and 5).

The wavefront reconstructed visually has better fidelity than the three patients when compared with the reference epicardial potential. The wavefront reconstructed by the patient is spread out as a round shape into the right ventricle (RV) when measurement noise increases. Thus, reconstructed potential mapping by the three patients could not reproduce the propagation shape of the parallel wave shown in the reference epicardial potential, thus, the conduction block can be detected in this region (see Fig. 3 up row).

From visual observation, the existence of fragmented, double, or multiphasic components are observed. The conduction block was shown by the data from 21 patients. The results of the remaining 2 patients show large areas. The potentials

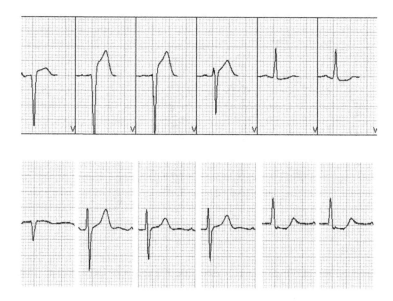

Fig. 3. Selected 6-lead signals of BSPM. Up row: input BSPM (processed). Bottom row: final TMP estimates. They are in close accordance with relative root mean squared error as 0.15.

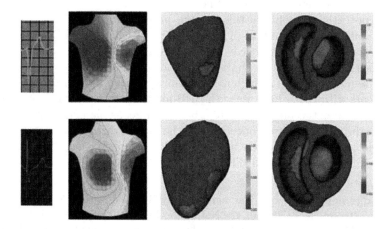

Fig. 4. Two cases: LBBB (up row) and RBBB (bottom row). For each row, the first figure is the input BSPM; the second figure is the mapping of BSPM on the thorax model; the third and fourth figures are the 3D visualization on the heart model from different angles.

distribution of conduction block spreads paralleled to the region near the cardiac apex, where the conduction block is terminated at the cardiac apex (Fig. 3 bottom row).

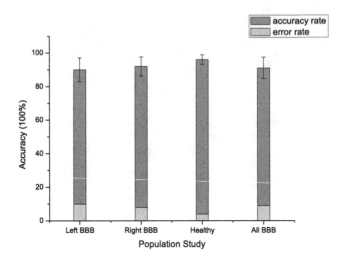

Fig. 5. The accuracy of our proposed system on the cases of BBB and normal cases.

4   Conclusions

In this chapter, we proposed a system in which the 3D transmembrane potential is estimated and visualized in the 3D heart model. Through the analysis of the epicardial potential mapping in this system, patients with BBB are easily and accurately distinguished instead of from empirically checking ECG. Therefore the diagnosis of BBB is improved using this system. Three-dimensional mapping is effective in the precise characterization of BBB in terms of the global activation sequence as well as regional duration, velocity, and functional behavior in patients with BBB. Patients with BBB may benefit from this non-invasive 3D epicardial potential mapping system before surgeons plan surgery.

For the future work, we concern that the personalized heart-torso model can be used instead of using one model for all patients. We can thus build the patient-specific system through this work.

Acknowledgement. This work was supported by National Natural Science Foundation of China (Grant No. 61301010), the Natural Science Foundation of Fujian Province (Grant No. 2014J05080), Research Fund for the Doctoral Program of Higher Education (20130121120045) and by the Fundamental Research Funds for the Central Universities (Grant No. 2013SH005).

References

1. Madias, J.E.: Left bundle branch block and suspected acute myocardial infarction. J. Electrocardiol. **46**(1), 11–12 (2013)
2. Taccardi, B., Punske, B., Lux, R., MacLEOD, R., Ershler, P., Dustman, T., Vyhmeister, Y.: Useful lessons from body surface mapping. J. Cardiovasc. Electrophysiol. **9**(7), 773–786 (1998)

3. Kors, J., van Herpen, G.: How many electrodes and where? a [ldquo] poldermodel [rdquo] for electrocardiography. J. Electrocardiol. **35**(4), 7–12 (2002)
4. Hisamatsu, K., Kusano, K., Morita, H., Takenaka, S., Nagase, S., Nakamura, K., Emori, T., Matsubara, H., Ohe, T.: Usefulness of body surface mapping to differentiate patients with brugada syndrome from patients with asymptomatic brugada syndrome. Acta Med. Okayama **58**(1), 29–36 (2004)
5. Wang, L., Wong, K.C.L., Zhang, H., Shi, P.: Noninvasive functional imaging of volumetric cardiac electrical activity: a human study on myocardial infarction. In: Metaxas, D., Axel, L., Fichtinger, G., Székely, G. (eds.) MICCAI 2008, Part I. LNCS, vol. 5241, pp. 1042–1050. Springer, Heidelberg (2008)
6. Donis, V., Guillem, M., Climent, A., Castells, F., Chorro, F., Millet, J.: Diagnosis of bundle branch block by analyzing body surface potential maps. In: Computers in Cardiology, 2008, pp. 97–100. IEEE (2008)
7. Aizawa, Y., Takatsuki, S., Sano, M., Kimura, T., Nishiyama, N., Fukumoto, K., Tanimoto, Y., Tanimoto, K., Murata, M., Komatsu, T., et al.: Brugada syndrome behind complete right bundle-branch block. Circulation **128**(10), 1048–1054 (2013)
8. Donis, V., Guillem, M., Climent, A., Castells, F., Chorro, F., Millet, J.: Improving the diagnosis of bundle branch block by analysis of body surface potential maps. J. Electrocardiol. **42**(6), 651–659 (2009)
9. Auricchio, A., Fantoni, C., Regoli, F., Carbucicchio, C., Goette, A., Geller, C., Kloss, M., Klein, H.: Characterization of left ventricular activation in patients with heart failure and left bundle-branch block. Circulation **109**(9), 1133–1139 (2004)
10. Stenroos, M., Haueisen, J.: Boundary element computations in the forward and inverse problems of electrocardiography: comparison of collocation and Galerkin weightings. IEEE Trans. Biomed. Eng. **55**(9), 2124–2133 (2008)
11. Wang, L., Qin, J., Wong, T., Heng, P.: Application of l1-norm regularization to epicardial potential reconstruction based on gradient projection. Phys. Med. Biol. **56**, 6291 (2011)
12. Desai, A., Yaw, T., Yamazaki, T., Kaykha, A., Chun, S., Froelicher, V.: Prognostic significance of quantitative qrs duration. Am. J. Med. **119**(7), 600–606 (2006)
13. Maynard, S., Menown, I., Manoharan, G., Allen, J., McC Anderson, J., Adgey, A.: Body surface mapping improves early diagnosis of acute myocardial infarction in patients with chest pain and left bundle branch block. Heart **89**(9), 998–1002 (2003)

Confidence Weighted Local Phase Features for Robust Bone Surface Segmentation in Ultrasound

Niamul Quader[1]([✉]), Antony Hodgson[2], and Rafeef Abugharbieh[1]

[1] Department of Electrical and Computer Engineering,
The University of British Columbia, Vancouver, BC, Canada
{niamul,rafeef}@ece.ubc.ca
[2] Department of Mechanical Engineering, The University of British Columbia,
Vancouver, BC, Canada
ahodgson@mech.ubc.ca

Abstract. Ultrasound (US) image guidance in orthopaedic surgery is emerging as a viable non-invasive alternative to the currently dominant radiation-based modalities. Though it offers many advantages including reduced imaging costs and safer operation, the relatively low US image quality complicates data processing and visualization. We propose a novel approach for robust bone localization that integrates multiple US image features including local phase information, local signal attenuation, and bone shadowing to robustly segment bone surfaces. We demonstrate the advantages of our approach in different contexts including improved segmentation quality, increased registration accuracy, and decreased sensitivity to parameter setting. We present quantitative and qualitative validation on a bovine femur phantom and on real-life clinical pelvis US data from 18 trauma patients using computed tomography (CT) image sets as ground truth.

Keywords: Ultrasound · Local phase features · Shadowing effect · Confidence map · Orthopaedic imaging · Segmentation · Bone imaging

1 Introduction

Ultrasound (US) bone imaging is receiving increasing attention in computer assisted orthopaedic surgery (CAOS) applications. The primary motivation is reducing the use of ionizing radiation based modalities (X-ray/CT), which would lead to safer real-time imaging. This trend has the potential to impact a wide range of applications in orthopaedics. For example, tracked US could improve navigation of pedicle screw placement [1]. Intraoperative US could also supplement fluoroscopy-based procedures, such as pelvic fracture fixation [2, 3]. In pediatric orthopaedics, Cheung et al. [4] demonstrated the potential benefits of US imaging in routine checkups of scoliosis patients. Furthermore, in spine imaging, US bone surface extraction was shown to be promising for needle-insertion applications [5].

Bone surface extraction based on the detection of symmetric response features was recently shown to be a powerful approach [6, 7]. However, local symmetry features

© Springer International Publishing Switzerland 2014
M.G. Linguraru et al. (Eds.): CLIP 2014, LNCS 8680, pp. 76–83, 2014.
DOI: 10.1007/978-3-319-13909-8_10

remain prone to false detection of soft-tissue interfaces that often exhibit features similar to those of bone. Furthermore, though quite effective on relatively flat (i.e. sparsely-oriented) structures, raw phase symmetry responses require tedious non-intuitive parameter tuning procedures to correctly identify complex bone shapes. Attempts to automate the parameter selection process have been made [7] but persistent false positives remain, especially at soft tissue interfaces. Apart from approaches based on local symmetry features, other bone-surface segmentation methods exist that exploit the bone shadowing effect and local image intensity. Foroughi et al. [8] used dynamic programming on intensity and local gradient information to segment bone contours in 2D images. The approach has shown adequate clinical accuracy in 2D US images, but it requires region-of-interest selection to remove soft-tissue interfaces near the skin surface and the method was only applied to 2D US images. Another bone contour detection scheme relied on depth weighted adaptive thresholding and subsequent morphological opening/closing operators to enhance segmented bone surfaces in 2D images [9]. A recent study used eigen-analysis information from a multi-scale 3D Hessian matrix to enhance sheet-like surfaces for the purpose of generating 3D segmentations of large bones [10]. However, results from these techniques remain heavily dependent on quality of the US image, as well as on the depth and complexity of the imaged bone due to the effects of shadowing and attenuation of local intensities.

Despite their aforementioned limitations, local image phase features were shown to be effective for bone segmentation in certain subsets of US images. We therefore hypothesized that identifying and integrating *additional* features of bone surfaces would increase robustness and accuracy of the segmentation. The first key feature we use is local phase symmetry (PS). As widely studied, bone surfaces in US typically exhibit ridge-like responses that are well captured by local image PS features [6]. To calculate those, we use a 3D log-Gabor filter as our quadrature filter since it can be constructed with arbitrary bandwidth. The second key feature of bone material that we use is its significantly higher US attenuation effect compared to other tissues, which results in the characteristic shadowing below the bone surface in the US image. To quantify this shadowing and attenuation feature, we employ Karamalis et al.'s [11] shadow detection algorithm, which extracts a transmission model for an US image. Finally, we combine the aforementioned features into a hybrid feature that we call confidence-in-phase-symmetry (CPS) and that is intended to augment the PS measure in regions where shadowing and attenuation is large. We limit our presentation to 3D due to space limitations and since a 2D version is a straight forward simplification that would instead use a 2D log-Gabor filter bank.

2   Methods

Given a 3D US volume, $I_{x,y,z}$, we first extract phase symmetry information, $PS_{x,y,z}$, using *uniformly oriented filters* (Sect. 2.1). To alleviate the challenging and time-consuming problem of precise tuning of filter parameters to reduce outliers, we supplement the PS measures using an attenuation metric, $A_{x,y,z}$, and a shadowing metric, $S_{x,y,z}$ (Sect. 2.2). We combine the three measures, $PS_{x,y,z}$, $A_{x,y,z}$ and $S_{x,y,z}$ (Sect. 2.3) to generate our hybrid feature, $CPS_{x,y,z}$.

2.1   Local Phase Symmetry Feature

Similar to [6], we calculate a 3D PS measure from even and odd symmetric log-Gabor filter responses, denoted e_{rm} and o_{rm}, respectively, compensated by a noise power threshold, T_r, over all scales r and all orientations, m, with ε being a small number to prevent division by zero:

$$PS = \frac{\sum_r \sum_m [[|e_{rm}| - |o_{rm}|]] - T_r}{\sum_r \sum_m \sqrt{e_{rm}^2 + o_{rm}^2} + \varepsilon}. \tag{1}$$

In the frequency domain, the 3D log-Gabor filter bank has the transfer function:

$$3DG = exp[\frac{(log(\omega/\omega_{0i}))^2}{2(log(k/\omega_{0i}))}] * exp(-\frac{\alpha(\varphi_j, \theta_j)^2}{2\sigma_\alpha^2}), \tag{2}$$

where subscripts i and j represent a scale and an orientation, respectively, of the filter bank. k is the standard deviation of the Gabor filter in the radial direction and ω_{0i} is the central frequency. $\alpha(\varphi_i, \theta_i)$ controls the 3D orientation of the filter where φ_i and θ_i are the azimuth and elevation angles, respectively, and σ_α determines the angular band-width. The log-Gabor function is scaled with constant ratio filters by keeping the term k/ω_{0i} constant and using multiples of a minimum wavelength, λ_{min}.

2.2   Attenuation and Shadowing Feature

Similar to Karamalis et al. [11] we calculate a confidence map to quantify both the attenuation and shadowing properties in US images. We run a random walk [12] to calculate virtual signal strengths at every pixel in each ultrasound slice, given a signal being transmitted from virtual transducer locations at the top of the image slice. Essentially, the virtual signal strength of a pixel is the probability of a random walk (starting from the pixel itself), to reach the virtual transducers, and is computed from the graph Laplacian matrix. For different combinations of two nodes, v_i and v_j, the graph Laplacian matrix is defined as:

$$L_{ij} = \begin{cases} d_i & if \quad i = j \\ -w_{ij} & if \quad v_i \; adjacent \; to \; v_j, \\ 0 & otherwise \end{cases} \tag{3}$$

where w_{ij} represent the edge weights and $d_i = \sum_j w_{ij}$ [12]. This Laplacian matrix, L, is reformulated and decomposed into blocks of marked nodes, M, and blocks of unmarked nodes, with B being an incident matrix:

$$L = \begin{bmatrix} L_M & B \\ B^T & L_U \end{bmatrix}. \tag{4}$$

The solution for the desired unknown probabilities of unmarked nodes X_U can be found using $L_U X_U = -B^T X_M$, where X_M represents the known unit probabilities at the seed-points [11]. The edge-weights, w_{ij}, are then assigned in the horizontal, vertical and diagonal direction: $w_{ij}^H = \exp(-\beta(|c_i - c_j| + \gamma))$, $w_{ij}^V = \exp(-\beta(|c_i - c_j|))$, $w_{ij}^D = \exp(-\beta(|c_i - c_j|))$. The term, $c_i = g_i \exp(-\alpha l_i)$, is the depth-based intensity gradient controlled by parameter α, and γ represents the penalty of a horizontal and diagonal walk compared to a vertical walk. β controls robustness of the overall result of random walk. However, β barely affects the resulting confidence maps between the range $\beta = 90$ to $\beta = 120$ [11].

In a 2D ultrasound image $I_{x,y}$, the confidence map, $m_{x,y}$, resulting from the abovementioned probability map, ranges between 0 and 1. The values can be interpreted as relative signal strengths at different image locations. We calculate a local attenuation measure, $A_{x,y}$, which has a value between 0 and 1:

$$A_{x,y} = \frac{\sum_w (m_{x,y} - m_{min})}{\max(\sum_w (m_{x,y} - m_{min}))}, \tag{5}$$

where w refers to 2D windows at multiple scales around $m_{x,y}$ of dimensions $\lambda_{min}/2$, $\lambda_{min}/4$ and $\lambda_{min}/6$, where λ_{min} is the lowest scale used in the PS calculation, and m_{min} is the corresponding minimum node values in the windows. $A_{x,y}$ tends to highlight bone surfaces due to the stronger reduction of signal strength, Δm, at the bone surface. Similarly, we measure a shadowing feature, $S_{x,y}$, which has a value between 0 and 1:

$$S_{x,y} = \frac{\sum_w m_{x,y}/(m_{min})}{\max[\sum_w m_{x,y}/(m_{min})]}, \tag{6}$$

which quantifies the shadowing effect at location (x, y). This feature is strong at points characterized by a relative deficiency in signal strength. Although $A_{x,y}$ and $S_{x,y}$ seem related, both are needed to better highlight bone surfaces. $A_{x,y}$ alone will tend to fail for deeper bone surfaces, whereas $S_{x,y}$ alone will tend to erroneously highlight US artifacts and noise below the actual bone surface.

Finally, we concatenate the responses measured in each 2D slice into 3D response images designated as $A_{x,y,z}$ and $S_{x,y,z}$. It is worth mentioning that a random walk in 3D may be more appropriate if the US transducer directly acquired 3D images. However, since our US transducer (Ultrasonix, 4DL14-5/38 Linear 4D) acquires a set of 2D images, separated spatially and temporally, we opted to initially use a 2D random walk for our experiments.

2.3   Combined Feature for Bone Surface Localization

To combine the features, we define the bone membership probability:

$$P_{x,y,z} = \begin{cases} a_1 * A_{x,y,z} + a_2 * S_{x,y,z} + a_3 * PS_{x,y,z} & \text{if } PS > 0 \\ 0 & \text{if } PS = 0 \end{cases}, \tag{7}$$

where a_1, a_2 and a_3 are weights. In our experimentation, we initially set each weight to 1/3. We defer the optimization of weights, a_1, a_2, a_3, for future work.

Along each column y in the metric, $P_{x,y,z}$, we identify the maximum value, and extract the corresponding voxel location, (x_m, y_m, z_m). These locations correspond to the highest bone surface membership confidence and thus can provide a more reliable bone segmentation mask. We evaluate the mean, μ, and the standard deviation, σ, of the confidence map values, $m(x_m, y_m, z_m)$, and formulate our final CPS feature as:

$$CPS_{x,y,z} = \begin{cases} P_{x,y,z} * PS_{x,y,z} & if \ |m_{x,y,z} - \mu| < \sigma \\ 0 & otherwise \end{cases} \tag{8}$$

Here, μ characterizes the statistical mean of the confidence map (or relative signal strength) values at the bone surface. We denote $\mu \pm \sigma$ to be the boundaries of the aforementioned mask. This formulation is based on the notion that the shadow just below the bone surface and the region just above the bone surface should ideally have similar patterns of confidence values, $m_{x,y,z}$.

3   Results and Discussion

To assess the performance of the CPS feature, we evaluated it on US image sets with corresponding CT data from an *ex-vivo* bovine femur phantom as well as from *in-vivo* pelvic data collected from 18 trauma patients (obtained as part of routine clinical care under appropriate institutional review board approval). We compare our proposed CPS method against a previously-reported version of PS [6]. The PS surface for both methods was based on empirical filter parameters set to values similar to those described in [6]: *scale* = 1, k/ω_{0i} = 0.25, λ_{min} = 25, σ_α = 15°, and *number of orientations* = 6. Also, similar to what was described in [11], we used α = 2, β = 90, and γ = 0.2, for generating the confidence map. Throughout our study, these selected parameters were not changed.

The *ex-vivo* bovine femur (Fig. 1(a)) was placed in a polyvinyl chloride-filled cylindrical tube, with fiducials added to enable a direct comparison between the US and CT-derived surfaces. The bovine phantom represents a cylindrical (multi-directional) structure. Using the CT-derived surface (Fig. 1(b)) as the ground truth, we observed that the CPS-based surface (Fig. 1(e)) was able to remove considerably more soft-tissue outliers compared to PS alone (Fig. 1(d)).

To quantify the accuracy of segmentation, we registered the two surfaces (US-derived and CT-derived) using the fiducial locations. We then calculated a surface registration error (SRE) as the Euclidean root mean square distance between the segmented bone surfaces from the registered US and CT datasets [13]. The CPS algorithm produced a SRE of 0.236 mm, vs 0.538 mm for PS alone (Fig. 2(a)).

For the *in-vivo* pelvic data, where we do not have access to fiducial markers, we used *automatic* Gaussian mixture model (GMM)-based registration [13] to align the CT- and US-derived bone surfaces and computed the corresponding surface registration error (SRE) or surface fitting error (SFE), therefore avoiding any biases related to

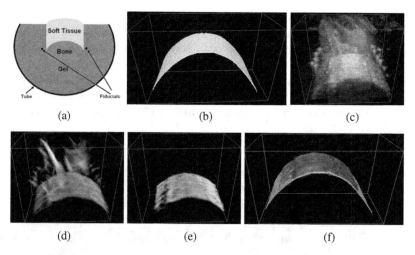

(a)   (b)   (c)

(d)   (e)   (f)

Fig. 1. Qualitative result on ex-vivo bovine femur data. (a) Bovine phantom setup, (b) CT volume showing segmented upper bone surface, (c) corresponding US volume, (d) PS, (e) proposed CPS, (f) overlay of segmented CT bone surface (orange) and extracted CPS based US bone surface (green) (Color figure in online).

any landmark selection. The final bone surfaces that were used during the registration algorithm were determined from the maximum of feature responses along the direction of US probe. Results are summarized in Fig. 2(b).

Figure 3 shows qualitative results of the CPS algorithm compared with two versions of the PS method, one using the empirical parameters described above and the other using optimized parameters determined as described in [7]. The optimization of parameters in [7, 13] relies on the assumption that bone surfaces will have the most significant ridge-like features in the ultrasound image, and performs a subsequent simplification of filter bank. Though successful in reducing soft-tissue outliers compared to empirical parameter-based PS, over-simplification may cause loss of true positives, as can be seen in the first example of Fig. 3. Also, note that some soft-tissue

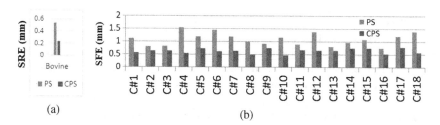

(a)   (b)

Fig. 2. Quantitative results. (a) Bovine phantom. Note that our proposed CPS based segmentation resulted in a 0.302 mm reduction in error compared to PS. (b) In-vivo pelvic data across all subjects (C#1 to C#18). Note that our proposed CPS resulted in a reduction in error which is significant at (p < 0.0002) based on Wilcoxon signed rank test compared to PS.

interfaces remain after optimized PS segmentation, since their response to the optimized filter bank is similar to that of bone surface. For both examples, the proposed CPS method appears to have improved bone surface segmentation, as illustrated in Fig. 3.

In terms of computational cost, for a 152 × 158 × 112 US volume, CPS required a small increase in run time with an average of 0.263 s per US slice, compared to 0.216 s for PS only. All tests were run on a Xeon(R) 3.40 GHz CPU computer with 8 GB RAM with MATLAB code.

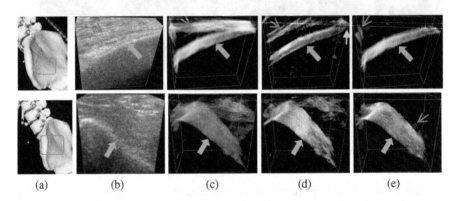

(a)   (b)   (c)   (d)   (e)

Fig. 3. Qualitative results: segmented bone surfaces around *in-vivo* pelvis, with two different US transducer locations and orientations. (a) Segmented CT with box representing approximate location of US transducer, (b) corresponding B-mode US volume, (c) PS based on empirical parameters, (d) PS based on optimized parameters [13], (e) proposed CPS feature based on augmented features with (b). Green arrows point to actual bone surfaces, red arrows point to soft-tissue interfaces, and the yellow arrow in the first example points to missing bone surface points. Our proposed CPS method appears to demonstrate qualitatively improved bone surface extraction and improved soft-tissue artifact reduction compared to both prior PS methods (Color figure in online).

4   Conclusions

We proposed a novel US bone enhancement algorithm that builds on PS-based bone segmentation by augmenting PS with certainty cues generated by a random walk. We demonstrated that this new feature enables better bone surface segmentation with minimal need for parameter tuning and can be computed with relatively little additional time. This method is simple to implement and provides an intuitive combination of complementary bone surface features and robustness to soft-tissue outliers. We validated the algorithm on a bovine phantom and on *in-vivo* clinical pelvic data, and both qualitative and quantitative results suggest promising robustness across a number of bone surface geometries; in contrast, phase symmetry seems to be primarily effective on relatively flat surfaces. In future work, we plan to evaluate the sensitivity of this metric to the choice of weights for the different features and to apply the CPS metric to additional scenarios of clinical interest.

References

1. Ungi, T., Moult, E., Schwab, J.H., Fichtinger, G.: Tracked ultrasound snapshots in percutaneous pedicle screw placement navigation: a feasibility study. Clin. Orthop. Relat. Res. **471**(12), 4047–4055 (2013)
2. Amin, D.V., Kanade, T., Digioia, A.M., Jaramaz, B.: Ultrasound registration of the bone surface for surgical navigation. J. Comput. Aided Surg. **8**(1), 1–16 (2003)
3. Tonetti, J., Carrat, L., Blendea, S.: Clinical results of percutaneous pelvic surgery: computer assisted surgery using ultrasound compared to standard fluoroscopy. J. Comput. Aided Surg. **6**(4), 204–211 (2001)
4. Cheung, C.W., Law, S.Y., Zheng, Y.P.: Development of 3D ultrasound system for assessment of adolescent idiopathic scoliosis (AIS): and system validation. In: Proceedings IEEE Conference on Engineering Medical Biology Society (2013)
5. Hacihaliloglu, I., Rasoulian, A., Rohling, R.N., Abolmaesumi, P.: Statistical shape model to 3D ultrasound registration for spine interventions using enhanced local phase features. In: Mori, K., Sakuma, I., Sato, Y., Barillot, C., Navab, N. (eds.) MICCAI 2013, Part II. LNCS, vol. 8150, pp. 361–368. Springer, Heidelberg (2013)
6. Hacihaliloglu, I., Abugharbieh, R., Hodgson, A.J., Rohling, R.: Bone segmentation and fracture detection in ultrasound using 3D local phase features. In: Metaxas, D., Axel, L., Fichtinger, G., Székely, G. (eds.) MICCAI 2008, Part I. LNCS, vol. 5241, pp. 287–295. Springer, Heidelberg (2008)
7. Hacihaliloglu, I., Guy, P., Hodgson A., Abugharbieh, R.: Volume-specific parameter optimization of 3D local phase features for improved extraction of bone surfaces in ultrasound images. Int. J. Med. Robot. Comput. Assist. Surg. (2013)
8. Foroughi, P., Boctor, E., Swatrz, M.J., Taylor, R.H., Fichtinger, G.: Ultrasound bone segmentation using dynamic programming. In: IEEE Ultrasonics Symposium, pp. 2523–2526 (2007)
9. Kowal, J., Amstutz, C., Langlotz, F., TAlib, H., Ballester, M.G.: Automated bone contour detection in ultrasound B-mode images for minimally invasive registration in computer assisted surgery an in vitro evaluation. Int. J. Med. Robot. Comput. Assist. Surg. **3**, 341–348 (2007)
10. Fanti, Z., Torres, F., Cosío, F.A.: Preliminary results in large bone segmentation from 3D freehand ultrasound. In: International Seminar on Medical Information Processing and Analysis (2013)
11. Karamalis, A., Wein, W., Klein, T., Navab, N.: Ultrasound confidence maps using random walks. Med. Image Anal. **16**, 1101–1112 (2012)
12. Grady, L.: Random walks for image segmentation. IEEE Trans. Pattern Anal. Mach. Intell. **28**, 1768–1783 (2006)
13. Hacihaliloglu, I., Brounstein, A., Guy, P., Hodgson, A., Abugharbieh, R.: 3D ultrasound-CT registration in orthopaedic trauma using GMM registration with optimized particle simulation-based data reduction. In: Ayache, N., Delingette, H., Golland, P., Mori, K. (eds.) MICCAI 2012, Part II. LNCS, vol. 7511, pp. 82–89. Springer, Heidelberg (2012)

Evaluation of Electromagnetic Tracking for Stereoscopic Augmented Reality Laparoscopic Visualization

Xinyang Liu[✉], Sukryool Kang, Emmanuel Wilson, Craig A. Peters, Timothy D. Kane, and Raj Shekhar

Sheikh Zayed Institute for Pediatric Surgical Innovation, Children's National Health System, Washington, DC, USA
{xliu,rshekhar}@childrensnational.org

Abstract. Without the requirement of line-of-sight, electromagnetic (EM) tracking is increasingly studied and used in clinical applications. We designed experiments to evaluate a commercial EM tracking system in three situations: using the EM sensor by itself; fixing the sensor onto the handle of a stereoscopic (i.e., 3D) laparoscope; and placing the sensor on the outside surface of the head of a laparoscopic ultrasound (LUS) transducer. The 3D laparoscope and the LUS transducer are core elements in our stereoscopic laparoscopic augmented reality visualization system, which overlays real-time LUS image on real-time 3D laparoscopic video for minimally invasive laparoscopic surgery. Jitter error, positional static and dynamic accuracies were assessed with the use of LEGO® basic bricks and building plates. The results show that the EM tracking system being tested yields satisfactory accuracy results and the attachment of the sensor to the planned positions on the probes is possible.

Keywords: Electromagnetic (EM) tracking · Augmented reality · Lapaoroscopic visualization

1 Introduction

Laparoscopic surgery is a minimally invasive alternative to conventional open surgery and has advantages that include improved outcomes, less scarring, and faster patient recovery. It has become the standard of care for certain surgical procedures such as cholecystectomy. Real-time video of the surgical field obtained using a laparoscopic camera is the primary imaging technique that guides laparoscopic surgeries currently. Despite the increasing application of laparoscopy to treat various pathologic conditions, visualization of the surgical field remains challenging. The majority of laparoscopes used in operating rooms (ORs) are two-dimensional (2D) and can provide only a relatively flat representation of three-dimensional (3D) anatomy and thus lack important depth cues. Moreover, although the current technology is able to provide intraoperative video with rich surface detail of the surgical anatomy, structures beneath the exposed organ

© Springer International Publishing Switzerland 2014
M.G. Linguraru et al. (Eds.): CLIP 2014, LNCS 8680, pp. 84–91, 2014.
DOI: 10.1007/978-3-319-13909-8_11

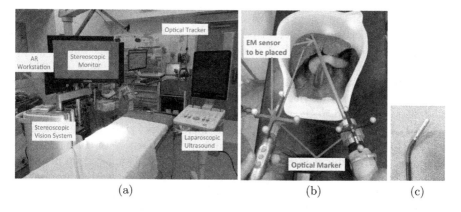

Fig. 1. (a): our current AR system based on optical tracking. (b): planned positions for embedding EM sensors (c): an example of the bending of the head of the LUS transducer.

surfaces, such as blood vessels and solid lesions, cannot be visualized in the video and might not be fully recognized by the operating surgeon during the surgery, causing avoidable medical complications.

Several groups [1–3] have reported augmented reality (AR) methods with the goal of enhancing intraoperative visualization of minimally invasive laparoscopic procedures. For laparoscopic surgeries, these methods overlay tomographic imaging data on intraoperative video to reveal internal anatomical structures not visible in the video images. Our group has built an AR system using a laparoscopic ultrasound (LUS) scanner (*flex* Focus 700, BK Medical, Herlev, Denmark), which is capable of seeing beneath the surface of organs in real time, for visualizing hidden structures [4,5]. To cope with inherent limitations of 2D cameras, our team has adopted stereoscopic (i.e., 3D) visualization (VSII, Visionsense Corp., New York, NY, USA), which is emerging now as a visualization option for laparoscopic surgeries. With the use of a commercial optical tracking system (Polaris, Northern Digital Inc., Waterloo, ON, Canada), we have further developed the capability to overlay real-time LUS data on real-time stereoscopic video accurately to provide 3D AR visualization without the prevailing problem of depth ambiguity. Figure 1(a) shows our current AR system based on optical tracking. Through successful demonstration of our AR system in animal and human studies, we have been gathering feedback from collaborating laparoscopic surgeons regarding the clinical feasibility and usefulness of the AR system. The feedback has focused on the use of optical tracking in a surgical setting. For our application, one limitation of using optical tracking is that the optical markers have to be placed outside the patient's body because of the line-of-sight requirement. For this, we designed a fixture to mount the optical markers on the handle of the LUS transducer (Fig. 1(b)). To maintain a rigid relationship between the marker and the LUS image, our current AR system does not allow four-way articulation (bending) of the imaging tip of the LUS transducer (Fig. 1(c)), which is a very desirable feature of the imaging device. In fact, a metallic cover is placed over the LUS transducer to prevent its tip from bending (Fig. 1(b)).

To incorporate this feedback of clinicians, we intend to replace optical tracking in our current AR system with electromagnetic (EM) tracking - a widely used real-time tracking technology without the line-of-sight restriction. We plan to embed an EM sensor on the tip of the LUS transducer (Fig. 1(b)) such that it can be allowed to bend freely and tracked. As with optical tracking, we intend to place an EM sensor on the handle of the 3D laparoscope, since it does not have a flexible tip and cannot be bent during surgery. The purpose of this study was to evaluate the tracking accuracy of a commercial EM tracking system made for OR-based applications. The result from this study will guide us in appropriately embedding EM sensors into the two imaging devices in the future.

In a typical EM tracking system, a field generator (FG) is used to create a local magnetic field of known geometry to localize positions and orientations of small sensors (diameter around 1 mm) inside the magnetic field. A thin wire is often required to connect the sensor to the control unit of the tracking system. In spite of many advantages over optical tracking, EM tracking is generally considered less accurate and less stable, especially when applied to clinical settings. This is mainly due to the fact that its magnetic field can be easily distorted by surrounding ferrous metals or conductive materials in the OR. These distortions affect the sensor position and orientation readings. Many investigations have focused on evaluating the accuracy of EM tracking systems in various environments. One common approach is to use a board phantom with drilled holes [6]. The distances among the holes are known (5 cm) and serve as the ground truth. Another popular method is the "scribbling" approach [7], in which sensor position data are collected by moving freely on a plane board with various elevations. A 180 mm^3 cube phantom with 225 holes of known geometry is introduced by Wilson et al. to measure position errors of EM tracking [8]. It is worth noting that several studies used inexpensive and easily available LEGO® basic bricks and building plate to design their experiments [7,9]. Moore et al.'s study [10] assessed EM tracking accuracy with the sensors embedded in a transesophageal echocardiography (TEE) probe. However, they did not take dynamic effects into account.

In general, errors of an EM tracking system can be classified into: (1) *static errors* - errors generated when the sensor is stationary for a certain period of time within the working volume of the FG - and (2) *dynamic errors* - errors generated when the sensor is moving or the environment is changing. For static errors, common measurements include precision, which measures jitter error (random noise); and accuracy, which measures exactness of relative positions. For each source of error, both positional and orientational errors can be measured. We designed our experiments to evaluate precision and both static and dynamic accuracies in three different situations: sensor by itself, and when the sensor is attached to the planned positions on the two imaging devices (Fig. 1(b)). Measurements in this study were restricted to positional errors.

2   Experimental Setup

A commercial EM tracking system with a 3.4 cm thick tabletop FG (Aurora, Northern Digital Inc., Waterloo, ON, Canada) was used in this study. Tabletop FG is specially designed for OR applications, and is supposed to be placed between the patient and the surgical table. The FG suppresses distortions caused by conductive or ferromagnetic materials located under it. Compatible 6 degrees of freedom (DoF) sensors (Aurora Catheter, Type 2; 1.3 mm diameter) were used for all experiments. In order to simulate a clinical setting, the tabletop FG was placed on a standard surgical table (Fig. 2(a)). In addition, the LUS machine and 3D laparoscopic visualization system were placed near the table.

A fixture to be fixed onto the handle of the 3D laparoscope was designed for our experiments (Fig. 2(b)). It is comprised of a cylindrical mount and a long straight bar with slots at 1 cm interval for placing the sensors. The diameter of the slot matched exactly the diameter of the sensor such that the sensor could be firmly fixed in the slot. Two sensors were placed, using tape, into the first

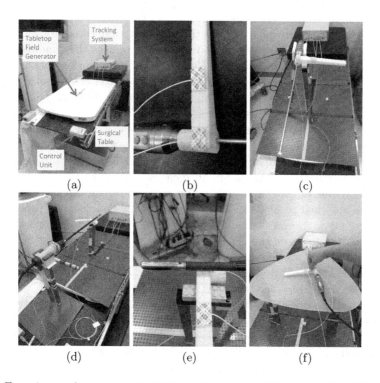

Fig. 2. Experiments for assessing the EM tracking system. (a): setup of the EM tracking system. (b): specially designed fixture with two EM sensors fixed on the handle of the 3D laparoscope. (c): setup to measure the static error with the 3D laparoscope turned on. (d): setup to measure the static error with the LUS transducer turned on. (e): EM sensor taped to the tip of the LUS transducer. (f): setup to measure the dynamic error with the 3D laparoscope turned on.

(i.e., the slot closest to the scope handle, and is referred to as the "First Sensor") and the fifth slot (referred to as the "Second Sensor"), respectively. The tips of the two sensors were exactly aligned with the edge of the fixture (Fig. 2(b)). Since the tracking system reports positions of the sensor tip, this sensor placement yielded a 5 cm distance between the two sensor tips, which was used as the ground truth for accuracy measurement.

If we denote a Cartesian coordinate system centered at the centroid of the surface of the tabletop FG (i.e., the centroid has coordinates $(0, 0, 0)$), the working volume of the FG can be expressed as (in mm) $x \in [-210, 210]$ (i.e., the width range of the FG), $y \in [-300, 300]$ (i.e., the length range of the FG), and $z \in [120, 600]$ (i.e., the height range above the FG). Note that the working volume of the FG we tested is in fact an ellipsoid-shaped volume, and thus, the sizes we refer to here are the maximum lengths in each dimension. We sampled the working volume with a total of 15 test points: 3 heights at $z = 25$ cm, 35 cm, and 45 cm; at each height, five points at coordinates $(0, 0), (0, -185), (0, 185), (-130, 0), (130, 0)$. It was less interesting for us to study positions with height below 25 cm, since in practice, our AR system is supposed to work with the patient lying on the tabletop FG.

We assessed the performance of EM tracking system in three situations: using the fixture (with two sensors) alone; fixing the fixture onto the handle of the 3D laparoscope (Fig. 2(b)); and stick the First Sensor to the surface of the head of the LUS transducer. For each situation, we measured jitter error, static accuracy and dynamic accuracy. Jitter error applies to single sensor, and in this case the one referred to as the First Sensor. Accuracy was obtained by comparing recorded distances between the two sensor tips to the 5 cm ground truth. To have consistent measurement of static errors, we aimed to position the tip of the First Sensor close to the target test point. This was achieved by utilizing LEGO® basic bricks and building plates. Six 10 inch by 10 inch plates were connected and taped on the surface of the FG. The fixture and the handles of the two probes were attached to LEGO®-made mounts using double-sided tapes. These mounts were elevated and positioned to the designated locations in a way such that the distance between the actual location of the tip of the First Sensor and the target test point was less than 5 mm. The Second Sensor maintained a fixed relative position to the First Sensor due to the rigid body of the fixture phantom. Figure 2(c) and (d) show the setup for measuring static errors when the fixture is attached to the working 3D laparoscope and LUS transducer, respectively. For easier positioning of the probes, two orientations of the probes (i.e., in Fig. 2(c) and (d), respectively) were used and kept (or held) consistently among different testing situations. As shown in Fig. 2(e), the First Sensor was stuck to the head of the LUS transducer using double-sided tape. The attachment location was selected to be the farthest location from the tip of the transducer, which could still yield bending of the transducer head.

Precision/jitter is defined, as the deviation of measured positions while one sensor is stationary for a certain period of time. At location x, it is calculated as the Root Mean Square (RMS) [11]

$$\text{Pre.}(x) = \sqrt{\frac{1}{N} \sum_{i=1}^{N} d(\bar{p}, p_i)^2}$$ (1)

where $d(\cdot, \cdot)$ is the Euclidean distance, and $\bar{p}$ is the mean position of N recorded positions p_i, $i = 1, \ldots, N$. The accuracy was calculated by

$$\text{Acc.}(x) = \frac{1}{N} \sum_{i=1}^{N} \left[d(p_i^1, p_i^2) - d_{\text{truth}} \right]$$ (2)

where p^1 and p^2 were recorded positions with regard to the First and the Second Sensor, respectively, and $d_{\text{truth}} = 5 \, \text{cm}$. For experiments of measuring static error, we recorded tracking for 20 s with a sampling interval of 1 s.

To measure dynamic errors, the fixture was moved freely with the operator's hand on a glass plate (Fig. 2(f)). The fixture was kept on the plate while moving. We tried to maintain a uniform speed of about 10 cm/s. Experiments were carried out for three situations same as above, and at three different heights (i.e., z = 25 cm, 35 cm, 45 cm). Tracking of the sensors were recorded for 30 s with a sampling interval of 1 s, and the accuracy was calculated using Eq. 2.

3   Result

The mean and maximum errors for three measurements in three situations are given in Table 1. The mean precision was calculated as the average of jitter errors (which was calculated using Eq. 1) at 15 locations. Similarly, the mean static accuracy is the mean of accuracies (calculated using Eq. 2) at 15 locations. The mean dynamic accuracy was the average accuracy over three heights. It should be noted that the maximum value in each case is not the maximum of instant values, but rather the maximum value (averaged according to Eq. 1 or Eq. 2) of 15 positions (for static) or 3 heights (for dynamic). For positions generating extreme values, e.g., 2.08 mm as the maximum static accuracy error for the case without the probe, we repeated the same experiments several times and took the mean value as the result. In a similar manner, errors grouped according to different heights are summarized in Table 2.

Table 1. Mean (maximum) errors for three different situations.

Situations	Jitter (mm)	Static accuracy (mm)	Dynamic accuracy (mm)
Sensor by itself	0.18 (0.49)	0.56 (2.08)	1.00 (1.43)
Attached to 3D probe	0.23 (0.69)	0.68 (1.12)	1.53 (2.12)
Attached to LUS probe	0.18 (0.57)	0.79 (1.72)	1.11 (1.61)

Table 2. Mean (maximum) errors at three different heights.

Height	Jitter (mm)	Static accuracy (mm)	Dynamic accuracy (mm)
25 cm	0.04 (0.05)	0.32 (0.70)	0.89 (1.10)
35 cm	0.13 (0.16)	0.80 (1.72)	1.03 (1.37)
45 cm	0.43 (0.69)	0.90 (2.08)	1.72 (2.12)

4   Discussion

The results we obtained in this study are consistent with results reported previously by other groups. Maier-Hein et al. [12] evaluated the same tracking system, i.e., *NDI Aurora* Tabletop FG, using standardized board phantom [6] with 5 cm distance as the ground truth. Our 0.56 mm static accuracy (without probe) lies between their reported laboratory accuracy (0.30 mm) and accuracy in a CT suite (0.90 mm), which is reasonable due to our simulated OR setting. In addition, Nafis et al. [7] assessed dynamic errors for a tabletop FG, i.e., 3D Guidance medSAFE™ Flat Transmitter (Ascension Technology, Shelburne, VT, USA), and they reported greater error with increased height from the FG, which is similar to what we have found. Besides these comparisons, we further noticed that the dynamic error is generally greater than the static error, which is as expected. Furthermore, the 0.23 mm jitter error when the sensor is attached to the 3D laparoscope is higher than the 0.18 mm error found in the other two situations.

Regarding incorporating EM tracking into our laparoscopic AR system, *NDI Aurora* Tabletop FG delivers satisfactory tracking accuracy according to our results, and is suitable for clinical applications due to its tabletop design. Although all three error measurements increase when the EM sensors are attached to either of the probes, the increased error is still acceptable. The evaluation results give us valuable insights for further embedding the EM sensors into the two probes. For 3D laparoscope, we could design a fixture similar as the one we used in this study but without the long straight bar, so that a sensor could be fixed at a location close to the handle of the probe. For LUS transducer, we intend to embed the sensor within the transducer head, approximately the same position as where we stuck the sensor in this work. The results from this study also suggest that the tracking system works better at lower heights, and this information is helpful to us in further design of our experiments for 3D camera and LUS calibration, as well as evaluation of the complete EM-tracked AR visualization system.

In conclusion, we have evaluated positional precision and accuracy, both statically and dynamically, for a commercial EM tracking system. The assessment experiments account for situations when just using the sensors alone and when they are attached to one of the two probes used in our stereoscopic laparoscopic AR visualization system. The results suggest that the tracking system has high accuracy and the attachment of the sensor to the planned positions on the probes is promising. These results will serve as the basis and benchmark and guide us in appropriately embedding the sensors into both imaging devices in our continued development of a superior laparoscopic visualization technology.

References

1. Marescaux, J., Rubino, F., Arenas, M., Mutter, D., Soler, L.: Augmented-reality-assisted laparoscopic adrenalectomy. JAMA **292**, 2214–2215 (2004)
2. Su, L.-M., Vagvolgyi, B.P., Agarwal, R., Reiley, C.E., Taylor, R.H., Hager, G.D.: Augmented reality during robot-assisted laparoscopic partial nephrectomy: toward real-time 3D-CT to stereoscopic video registration. Urology **73**(4), 896–900 (2009)
3. Liao, H., Inomata, T., Sakuma, I., Dohi, T.: 3-D augmented reality for mri-guided surgery using integral videography autostereoscopic image overlay. IEEE Trans. Biomed. Eng. **57**(6), 1476–1486 (2010)
4. Kang, X., Oh, J., Wilson, E., Yaniv, Z., Kane, T.D., Peters, C.A., Shekhar, R.: Towards a clinical stereoscopic augmented reality system for laparoscopic surgery. In: 2nd MICCAI Workshop on Clinical Image-based Procedures: Translational Research in Medical Imaging, Nagoya, Japan, pp 108–116 (2013)
5. Kang, X., Azizian, M., Wilson, E., Wu, K., Martin, A.D., Kane, T.D., Peters, C.A., Cleary, K., Shekhar, R.: Stereoscopic augmented reality for laparoscopic surgery. Surg. Endosc. **28**(7), 2227–2235 (2014)
6. Hummel, J.B., Bax, M.R., Figl, M.L., Kang, Y., Maurer, C., Birkfellner, W.W., Bergmann, H., Shahidi, R.: Design and application of an assessment protocol for electromagnetic tracking systems. Med. Phys. **32**(7), 2371–2371 (2005)
7. Nafis, C., Jensen, V., von Jako, R.: Method for evaluating compatibility of commercial elecromagnetic (EM) microsensor tracking systems with surgical and imaging tables. In: SPIE Medical Imaging: Visualization, Image-Guided Procedures and Modeling, San Diego, CA, pp. 69182 (2008)
8. Wilson, E., Yaniv, Z., Zhang, H., Nafis, C., Shen, E., Shechter, G., Wiles, A.D., Peters, T., Lindisch, D., Cleary, K.: A hardware and software protocol for the evaluation of electromagnetic tracker accuracy in the clinical environment: a multi-center study. In: SPIE Medical Imaging: Visualization, Image-Guided Procedures and Modeling, San Diego, CA, vol. 6509 (2007)
9. Haidegger, T., Fenyvesi, G., Sirokai, B., Kelemen, M., Nagy, M., Takács, B., Kovács, L., Benyó, B., Benyó, Z.: Towards unified electromagnetic tracking system assessment-static errors. In: Annual International Conference of the IEEE Engineering in Medicine and Biology Society, Boston, MA, pp. 1905–1908 (2011)
10. Moore, J.T., Wiles, A.D., Wedlake, C., Bainbridge, D., Kiaii, B., Trejos, A.L., Patel, R., Peters, T.M.: Integration of trans-esophageal echocardiography with magnetic tracking technology for cardiac interventions. In: SPIE Medical Imaging: Visualization, Image-Guided Procedures and Modeling, San Diego, CA, vol. 7625 (2010)
11. Much, J.: Error Classification and Propagation for Electromagnetic Tracking. Master Thesis, Technische Universität München, Munich, Germany (2008)
12. Maier-Hein, L., Franz, A.M., Birkfellner, W., Hummel, J., Gergel, I., Wegner, I., Meinzer, H.P.: Standardized assessment of new electromagnetic field generators in an interventional radiology setting. Med. Phys. **39**(6), 3424–3434 (2012)

Automatic Lung Tumor Segmentation with Leaks Removal in Follow-up CT Studies

Refael Vivanti[1]([⊠]), Onur A. Karaaslan[2],
Leo Joskowicz[1], and Jacob Sosna[2]

[1] The Rachel and Selim Benin School of Computer Science and Engineering,
The Hebrew University of Jerusalem, Jerusalem, Israel
refael.vivanti@mail.huji.ac.il, josko@cs.huji.ac.il
[2] Department of Radiology, Hadassah Hebrew University Medical Center,
Jerusalem, Israel

Abstract. We present a novel automatic algorithm for lung tumors segmentation in follow-up CT studies. The inputs are a baseline CT scan and a delineation of the tumors in it; the output is the tumor delineations in the follow-up scan. The algorithm consists of four steps: (1) deformable registration of the baseline and follow-up scans; (2) segmentation of the tumors in the follow-up scan; (3) geometry-based segmentation leaks correction; and (4) tumor boundary regularization. The key advantage of our method is that it automatically builds a patient-specific prior that increases segmentation accuracy and robustness and reduces observer variability. Our experimental results on 80 pairs of CT scans from 40 patients with ground-truth segmentations by a radiologist yield an average overlap error of 14.5 % (std = 5.6), a significant improvement from the 30 % (std = 13.3) result of stand-alone fast marching segmentation.

1 Introduction

Radiological follow-up of tumors is the cornerstone of modern oncology. Disease progression and response to treatment are routinely evaluated by measuring the tumor volume in a series of volumetric scans. Today, most radiologists rely on standards such as RECIST to estimate the tumor mass. It is well known that this estimate can be off by as much as 50 %. Previous research shows that true volumetric measurements are the most accurate information for tumor monitoring [1].

Tumor delineation is the main bottleneck of tumor volume computation. Manual delineation is time-consuming, is user-dependent, and requires expert knowledge. Semi-automatic segmentation methods, e.g., live wire and region growing, also require user interaction and may lead to large intra- and inter- observer variability. Automatic tumor segmentation poses significant challenges and is used in the clinic for only a handful of tumor types. Model-based methods are also limited, as they require a generic tumor prior. Moreover, most methods process each scan independently without considering that it is the same patient. Recent works show that using the baseline delineation as a patient-specific prior may improve robustness and accuracy [2].

In this paper we present a new, fully automatic algorithm for lung tumor segmentation in follow-up CT studies. The inputs are the baseline scan, the tumor's

© Springer International Publishing Switzerland 2014
M.G. Linguraru et al. (Eds.): CLIP 2014, LNCS 8680, pp. 92–100, 2014.
DOI: 10.1007/978-3-319-13909-8_12

delineations, and the follow-up CT scan; the outputs are the tumor's delineations in the follow-up CT scan. The baseline delineation can be obtained by semi-automatic segmentation methods. The algorithm consists of four steps: (1) deformable registration of the baseline and follow-up scans; (2) segmentation of the tumors in the follow-up CT scan using statistical intensity models; (3) detection and removal of tumors segmentation leaks using geometry-based methods for both the tumor and the adjacent anatomy and; (4) tumor boundary regularization to correct the partial volume effects.

The three most relevant research areas to our work are: (1) lung follow-up studies; (2) lung tumor segmentation, and (3) lung scans registration. We briefly discuss each next.

Hollensen et al. [3] address the task of follow-up studies of lung tumors. Their method starts with manual rough positioning followed by rigid registration. The baseline delineation is then used as the initialization of the follow-up segmentation by electric flow lines and min graph-cut. Their method, which is the closest to ours, is demonstrated on a small database of 10 cases and does not handle segmentation leaks.

Lung nodules segmentation and follow-up has received significant attention. It is usually easier than lung tumors due to known diameter and spherical shape. The VOLCANO'09 lung nodules follow-up challenge [4] comprises 13 groups and 50 datasets. Among the participating groups, Kostis et al. [5] present a method based on thresholding. Segmentation leaks to vessels are corrected with morphological opening adjusted by the user. Pleural surface attachments are removed with a separating plane, which is not adequate for larger tumors. Jirapatnakul et al. [6] model the pleural surface with a parabola for leaks removal. While this leak removal method is similar to ours, their nodule-specific heuristics may not always work for lung tumors.

Methods for individual stand-alone pulmonary tumors segmentation include thresholding, region growing, and level-sets. For PET/CT scans, Gribben et al. [7] propose to use the PET scan for tumor detection, followed by unsupervised Maximum A Posterior Markov Random Field on the registered CT scan values. Kanakatte et al. [8] also use the PET scan for tumor detection, but combine thresholding and components analysis to produce the final segmentation. Plajer et al. [9] classify lung tumors in standalone CT scans into five categories and apply mixed internal/external force segmentation and clustering. Awad et al. [10] use multi-parameter level-set with a sphere shape prior. Their validation on 21 tumors yields a volume overlap error of 30 %, which is excessive for disease progression evaluation.

Lungs CT scans registration is challenging because the lungs deformations are non-rigid. The EMPIRE10 lungs registration challenge [11] comprises 24 groups and 30 datasets. The highest scoring method by Song et al. [12] uses topology-preserving diffeomorphic transformations. Lung registration methods usually produce good results for the lungs, but may incur in large errors when used for tumor registration.

Our method has the following advantages over existing ones: (1) it is fully automatic; (2) it builds a strong patient-specific prior from the baseline tumor delineation that improves segmentation robustness and accuracy; (3) it performs local deformable registration to model more accurately the tumor transformation; (4) it corrects for tumor segmentation leaks with a new method based on the pulmonary surface geometry, and; (5) it accounts for segmentation errors resulting from the partial volume effect. Our experimental results on CT scans from 40 patients with ground-truth segmentations generated by a radiologist yields an average overlap error of 14.5 % (std = 4.1), a significant improvement of the 30 % (std = 13.3) of stand-alone level-set segmentation.

2 Method

The basic premise of our method is that the tumor delineation in the baseline scan is a high-quality prior for the follow-up scans. The algorithm consists of four steps.

2.1 Deformable Registration of the Baseline and the Follow-up Scans

The initial step is to register the baseline CT scan with the follow-up scan. This transformation defines the approximate location of the tumor mass in the follow-up and is used to build intensity priors to delineate the tumor in the follow-up scan.

We start by performing a deformable registration between the baseline and follow-up scans in the automatically detected lungs Region of Interest (ROI). This global lung ROI deformable registration consists of a rigid affine registration followed by a deformable registration with B-Splines. This stage usually registers the lungs properly, although the tumor itself may be poorly registered.

To overcome this challenge, we perform a separate local deformable registration for each tumor. The baseline tumor delineation is enclosed in a bounding ROI. The follow-up ROI is determined from the baseline tumor by projecting it to the follow-up scan using the global transformation and with an added margin. This local registration has three stages: (1) a pure translation registration to account for large changes in the tumor volume; (2) a rigid affine registration, and; (3) a deformable registration.

2.2 Initial Follow-up Tumor Segmentation

The segmentation is performed using a statistical model of the foreground (tumor) and the background (other structures). The foreground voxels are from the prior in the follow-up scan; the background voxels are from the prior neighborhood. Since the registration is not accurate, the foreground voxels may include background voxels and vice versa. To remove them, we classify the voxels into the two classes with the k-means algorithm and remove the class representing the registration error. For the foreground, we remove the class with the lower mean and vice versa. Next, we estimate Gaussians parameters to compute the initial tumor segmentation by Maximum Likelihood Estimation. Finally, we use morphological closing to remove small holes.

2.3 Segmentation Leaks Removal

Since the tumors may be attached to neighboring structures with similar intensities, any intensity-based segmentation method will include parts of these structures in the result. Our goal is to automatically detect these *segmentation leaks* [13], and correct them. For this, we use geometric models for the tumor and background structures.

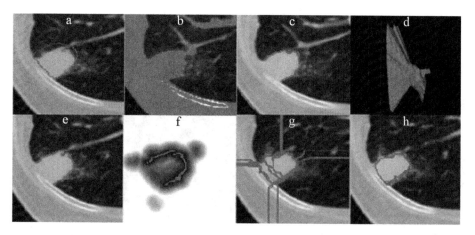

Fig. 1. Illustration of the segmentation process stages: (a) the baseline tumor delineation (red) overlaid on the corresponding follow-scan CT slice after registration; (b) maximum likelihood follow-up tumor segmentation (red) with leaks; (c) segmentation boundary B (red) as seen from the center point; (d) 3D view of the ray casting result; (e) follow-up tumor boundary (red) after leaks removal; (f) distance map from follow-up tumor boundary (red); (g) watershed regions, and; (h) final follow-up tumor segmentation (Color figure online).

We handle segmentation leaks to neighboring vessels, to the pleural wall, and/or to the diaphragm. Note that we cannot use the baseline shape as a prior, as it can change dramatically during the tumor growth/shrinkage. We automatically detect and correct the segmentation leaks in two stages. The first stage handles bottleneck-shaped leaks; the second stage handles leaks caused by missing boundaries.

In the first stage, we model the tumor as a star-shaped structure; i.e. structures for which there is a point from which the entire tumor boundary is visible. Empirically, we observe that the majority of lung tumors are star-shaped. We use our previous method for the detection and removal of bottleneck-shaped leaks [14]. The input to this step is the initial tumor segmentation with leaks and a point c in the segmented tumor kernel. We choose this point as the closest point to the center-of-mass in the segmentation prior. We perform dense ray casting to find the boundary of the tumor that is visible from c. We project a ray from c in all 3D directions, and record the voxel just before the ray leaves the segmentation volume as part of the segmentation boundary. The result is the segmentation boundary as seen from c.

The small segmentation leaks are detected as follows. When casting rays from the tumor center outwards, the rays will stop at a sharp boundary segments but will continue for the fuzzy/missing boundary segments, causing a segmentation leak. Consequently, the boundary of leak will not be connected to the tumor boundary, resulting in a discontinuity. In 3D, the actual tumor boundary will form a single connected component regardless of the number of leaks. To remove these leaks, we perform a connected components analysis on B and select the largest connected component that surrounds c to be the segmentation *known boundary*. The missing boundaries (holes) in this *known boundary* are the leaks. They are then removed by filling the boundary holes. To fill the holes, we first compute the voxels Euclidean

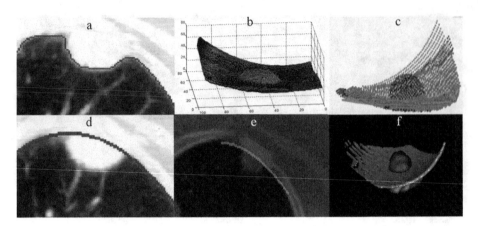

Fig. 2. Illustration of the background geometric modeling stages: (a) background and foreground boundary points (red) on a slice; (b) 3D model of the boundary points; (c) RANSAC result: green, parabolic surface, blue, inliers, red, outliers; (d) one slice with parabolic surface; (e) segmentation results: red, tumor, yellow, parabolic surface, green, leak; (f) 3D visualization (Color figure online).

distance map from the known boundary. Next, we identify the watershed regions in this distance map. Finally, we choose regions whose intersection with the known segmentation is greater than a predefined threshold. A voxel belongs to the known segmentation if it is on a ray connecting the center point c and a point in the known boundary (Fig. 1).

In the second stage we treat missing tumor boundaries. we use a parabolic surface as a local geometric model of the adjacent structures to determine it. This boundary shape is similar to the way a human delineator would complete the missing boundary, and it holds for the pleural surface, the diaphragm, and parts of the heart walls. We empirically found that this is better than using shape prior, e.g. as described in [10].

To create this model, we use the tumor segmentation of the previous stage and find its boundary points. These boundary points can be inliers from the adjacent structures borders or outliers from the tumor or vessels. We apply the RANSAC outlier detection framework with a parabolic surface model to simultaneously find the parabolic surface parameters and the outliers. We require the cloud of points to be monotonic in the z axis direction. To achieve this, we first rotate the cloud of points so that its axis of smallest variance, obtained from Principal Component Analysis (PCA), is aligned with the z axis. Next we fit a parabolic model to the resulting points cloud.

In RANSAC, we repeatedly choose six random points. We estimate the parabolic surface parameters from the points and use it to find which points are inliers. Finally, we choose the parabolic surface with the largest set of inliers. The final refinement step iteratively estimates the parabolic surface parameter using the inliers points. The iterations stop when inliers set size remains the same. Finally, we remove the part of the tumor that is separated from the center c by the parabolic surface (Fig. 2).

2.4   Tumor Boundary Refinement

The last step addresses the partial volume effect (PVE). The PVE results in blurred tumors boundaries that may cause variability in the tumor delineation by different radiologists and segmentation algorithms. To reduce this variability, we generate several possible segmentations and choose the best one. First, we compute the variance map of the image from the variance of a small window around each voxel. Then, we compute several segmentations by incrementally dilating or eroding by one voxel the tumor segmentation. We then compute for each such alternative segmentation the mean variance of its boundary voxels using the variance map and choose the one with the highest mean variance. This reduces the variability between different segmentations of the same tumor in different scans and/or different observers.

Table 1. Experimental results of 40 forward cases and 40 backwards cases. VOE: Volume Overlap Error, in %. ASSD: Average Symmetric Surface Distance in mm. Ours: our method; FM: Fast Marching method.

	Forward VOE		Forward ASSD		Backwards VOE		Reversed ASSD	
	Ours	FM	Ours	FM	Ours	FM	Ours	FM
Mean	14.47	26.84	1.03	2.73	15.37	33.28	1.03	4.32
Std	4.14	7.63	0.55	1.56	6.79	16.54	0.62	3.57
Min	6.32	14.86	0.17	0.69	6.35	12.72	0.33	0.65
Max	23.25	44.20	2.46	8.54	38.37	82.10	3.07	16.09

3   Experimental Results

We have evaluated our method on a database of CT scans from 40 patients. The scans were acquired on a 64-row CT scanner (Phillips Brilliance 64) and are of size $512 \times 512 \times 350$–500 voxels, with spatial resolution of 0.6–1.0×0.6–1.0×0.7–3 mm, with contrast agent administration. The cases were carefully chosen from the hospital archive by the radiologist co-author to represent the variety of patient ages, conditions, and pathologies. The mean time between the baseline and the follow-up scans is 4.9 months with Standard Deviation (std) of 2.4 months. The mean tumor volume is 43.8 ml with STD of 49.9 ml, and the mean volumetric change is 17.8 ml with STD of 29.7 ml. Of the 40 scans, 32 scans include tumors adhered to the lung wall and 8 have isolated tumors. An expert radiologist produced ground-truth delineations of the tumors in both the baseline and follow-up CT scans.

For the evaluation, we use each pair of scans twice: forward (from baseline to follow-up) and backwards (from follow-up to baseline). Although the backwards direction is not a real clinical case and is correlated to the pair in the forward direction, it provides additional data and attests the robustness and accuracy of our method. We present the results for the forward and backwards pairs separately to prevent bias.

We compare the results of our method with the ground-truth by computing the standard DICE volumetric overlap error (VOE) and the average symmetric surface distance (ASSD). For the B-spline, we chose a grid spacing of 12 mm. For the watershed region selection, we set the threshold to 10 %. We set the RANSAC iterations bound to 10,000, with a threshold of 3 voxels. We use 9 segmentations for VOE regularization with a $5 \times 5 \times 5$ window around each voxel.

We compare the results of our method to the fast marching segmentation method [14]. Fast marching requires a seed that serves as the center of the ground truth tumor segmentation. For the propagation speed function, we chose the inverted (minus) gradients map values. Since each iteration may yield a different segmentation, we stop the propagation when 90 % of the ground true was segmented. Note that although we use the fast marching method without a shape prior, we obtain similar or better results than other state-of-the-art methods that use fast marching or level sets with shape prior. For example, Awad et al. [10] report similar error measures to those we obtained with the generic fast marching method. Note that we "help" the fast marching method by using the ground truth for both seeding and for the termination criterion: without them, the results of the fast marching algorithm would probably be worse.

Table 1 summarizes the results. Our method reduced the VOE and standard deviation from 30 % (std = 13.3) for the level set method to 14.9 % (std = 5.6), an improvement of 50.4 % (std 57.5 %). It reduced the ASSD and standard deviation from 3.5 mm (std = 2.88) for the level-set method to 1 mm (std = 0.59), an improvement of 71.4 % (std 79.5 %). The minimum and maximum values were significantly improved. The minimum VOE was reduced from 14.86 % to 6.32 %, an improvement of 57 %. The minimum ASSD was reduced from 0.69 mm to 0.17 mm, an improvement of 75 %. The maximum VOE was reduced from 44.2 % to 23.25 %, an improvement of 47 %. The maximum ASSD was reduced from 8.54 mm to 2.46 mm, an improvement of 71 %. When we manually selected the best stopping threshold for each case, the fast marching method results were VOE of 26.2 % (std = 8.4) and ASSD of 1.4 mm (std = 1.6).

To quantify the contribution of the segmentation step, we compute the accuracy of the patient-specific prior, which can also be interpreted as the registration error in terms of the Volume Overlap Error. The VOE and ASSD after step 1 are 35.8 % (std = 17.6) and 4.3 mm (std = 6.6) respectively. This can be considered as a good registration result, but cannot serve as the final segmentation result since it is more than twice the final segmentation.

To quantify the contribution of the patient-specific prior, we left out the baseline scan and tumor's delineations and performed segmentation alone with the prior as a sphere of radius 30 voxels centered at the center of mass of the tumor ground truth. The segmentation failed in 8 out of 80 cases, and yielded VOE and ASSD errors of 18.6 % (std = 7.3) and 1.27 mm (std = 0.9) respectively for the other 72 cases. We conclude that both the patient-specific baseline prior and the local deformable baseline tumor registration are key to achieving accuracy and robustness.

4   Conclusion

We have presented a new automatic lung tumor segmentation method for follow-up CT studies. The inputs to the method are baseline CT scan of the lungs with delineation of the tumor, and a follow-up scan. A cascade of registration methods are used to transform the delineation into the follow-up scan. A statistical method then uses this prior to produce initial segmentation. A two-stage automatic segmentation leaks detection and removal use geometrical models of the foreground and background. The final step reduces the tumor boundaries variability caused by the partial volume effect by variation analysis.

The novelty of our work is in the use of patient specific model for the segmentation prior. This improves robustness by creating patient-specific statistical models of the tumors and the background. This observation is supported by an experiment in which the segmentation step was used with a weak sphere shape prior. The failure rate was 10 % instead of 0 % and the error rate was 25 % higher. Our registration method includes an additional tumor-specific local deformable registration step which refines the model prior. The segmentation leaks removal step relies on anatomic geometric constraints on the tumor and the adjacent structures. This geometric knowledge cannot be integrated in classic active contours methods, which may fail on large leaks. The modeling of the adjacent structures as a parabolic surface simulates the way a human would complete the missing boundary between the structures. The final step addresses the delineation variability caused by the PVE. Our results on 40 pairs of CT scans, each used forward and backwards, show a significant improvement over the fast marching method and may provide relevant clinical measurements for lung tumors. We plan to apply the proposed method to other organ segmentations from various imaging modalities.

References

1. Tuma, S.R.: Sometimes size does not matter: reevaluating RECIST and tumor response rate endpoints. J. Nat. Cancer Inst. **98**, 1272–1274 (2006)
2. Weizman, L., Ben-Sira, L., Joskowicz, L., Precel, R., Constantini, S., Ben-Bashat, D.: Automatic segmentation and components classification of optic pathway gliomas in MRI. In: Jiang, T., Navab, N., Pluim, J.P., Viergever, M.A. (eds.) MICCAI 2010, Part I. LNCS, vol. 6361, pp. 103–110. Springer, Heidelberg (2010)
3. Hollensen, C., Cannon, G., Cannon, D., Bentzen, S., Larsen, R.: Lung tumor segmentation using electric flow lines for graph cuts. In: Campilho, A., Kamel, M. (eds.) ICIAR 2012, Part II. LNCS, vol. 7325, pp. 206–213. Springer, Heidelberg (2012)
4. Reeves, A., Jirapatnakul, A.C.: The VOLCANO'09 MICCAI Challenge: Preliminary results. In: VOLCANO'09, pp. 353–364 (2009)
5. Kostis, W.J., et al.: Three-dimensional segmentation and growth-rate estimation of small pulmonary nodules in helical CT images. Trans. Med. Imag. **22**(10), 1259–1274 (2003)
6. Jirapatnakul, A.C., et al.: Segmentation of juxtapleural pulmonary nodules using a robust surface estimate. Int. J. Biomed. Imag. 1–14 (2011)
7. Gribben, H., et al.: MAP-MRF segmentation of lung tumours in PET/CT images. IEEE Int. Symp. Biomed. Imag. 290–293 (2009)
8. Kanakatte, A., et al.: A pilot study of automatic lung tumor segmentation from Positron Emission Tomography images using standard uptake values. Comp. Intel. Imag. Sig. Proc. 363–368 (2007)

9. Plajer, I.C., Richter, D.: A new approach to model based active contours in lung tumor segmentation in 3D CT image data. Inf. Tec. App Biomed. 1–4 (2010)

10. Awad, J., et al.: Three-dimensional lung tumor segmentation from x-ray computed tomography using sparse field active models. Med. Phys. **39**(2), 851–865 (2012)

11. Murphy, K., et al.: Evaluation of registration methods on thoracic CT: The EMPIRE10 Challenge Trans. Med. Imag. **30**(11), 1901–1920 (2011)

12. Song, G., Tustison, N.: Lung CT image registration using diffeomorphic transformation models. Med. Image Anal. Clinic 23–32 (2010)

13. Kronman, A., Joskowicz, L., Sosna, J.: Anatomical structures segmentation by spherical 3D ray casting and gradient domain editing. In: Ayache, N., Delingette, H., Golland, P., Mori, K. (eds.) MICCAI 2012, Part II. LNCS, vol. 7511, pp. 363–370. Springer, Heidelberg (2012)

14. Bærentzen, J.A.: On the implementation of fast marching methods for 3D lattices. Math. Model **13**, 1–19 (2001)

Patient Specific Simulation for Planning of Cochlear Implantation Surgery

Sergio Vera[1,2](✉), Frederic Perez[2], Clara Balust[2], Ramon Trueba[2],
Jordi Rubió[2], Raul Calvo[2], Xavier Mazaira[2], Anandhan Danasingh[3],
Livia Barazzetti[5], Mauricio Reyes[5], Mario Ceresa[4], Jens Fagertum[6],
Hans Martin Kjer[6], Rasmus Paulsen[6], and Miguel Ángel González Ballester[4,7]

[1] Computer Vision Center, UAB, Bellaterra, Spain
sergio.vera@cvc.uab.es
[2] Alma IT Systems, Barcelona, Spain
[3] MED-EL GMBH, Wien, Austria
[4] Universitat Pompeu Fabra, Barcelona, Spain
[5] Universitat Bern, Bern, Switzerland
[6] Denmark Technische Universitet, Lyngby, Denmark
[7] ICREA - Catalan Institution for Research and Advanced Studies, Barcelona, Spain

Abstract. Cochlear implantation is a surgical procedure that can restore the hearing capabilities to patients with severe or complete functional loss. However, the level of restoration varies highly between subjects and depends on patient-specific factors. This paper presents a software application for planning cochlear implantation procedures that includes patient-specific anatomy estimation using high resolution models, implant optimization for patient-specific implant selection, simulation of mechanical and electrical properties of the implant as well as clinical reporting.

Keywords: Cochlear implant · Patient specific · Simulation · Planning

1 Introduction

A Cochlear Implant (CI) is a sound-to-electrical transducer device that can restore hearing to patients suffering hearing impairment, a condition affecting over 24 % of the population worldwide [12]. Cochlear Implants consist of a speech processor which performs filtering of the audio signal to improve the hearing of specific frequencies, and a sub-cutaneous transductor and an Electrode Array (EA) that is inserted into the cochlea and can stimulate the auditory nerve fibers, bypassing the damaged hair cells (Fig. 1).

Cochlear implantation surgery requires to gain access to the inner ear, to make the cochlea accessible, by drilling the temporal bone behind the ear. The target structure is small and the access through the middle ear is close to delicate

Miguel A. Gonzalez Ballester: This research has been funded by the European Union FP7 grant agreement no. HEAR-EU 304857.

© Springer International Publishing Switzerland 2014
M.G. Linguraru et al. (Eds.): CLIP 2014, LNCS 8680, pp. 101–108, 2014.
DOI: 10.1007/978-3-319-13909-8_13

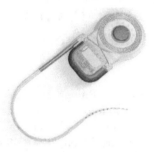 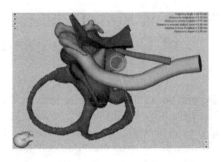

Fig. 1. (Left: Sub-cutaneal part of the cochlear implant with the transductor and electrode array. Right: Segmentation of structures of the middle and inner ear: Cochlea and semicircular canals (red) ossicles (purple), external auditory canal (blue), facial nerve (yellow) and chorda timpany (orange) (Color figure online).

structures such as the ossicles, chorda tympani and facial nerve. Careful planning of the access path considering the risk areas, is the element that decides if the electrode insertion will be performed through the membrane that covers the round window of the cochlea or through a hole drilled into the cochlea (cochleostomy). In this complex scenario, a planning software can help the surgeon to estimate the risks of the intervention and choose the best approach. Extreme care has to be taken during the insertion of the electrode array inside the cochlea. The depth and angle of insertion has to be the adequate to provide improved hearing without jeopardizing residual hearing capabilities. This is because the cochlear inner structures are delicate, and can be damaged easily by an incorrect insertion procedure. It follows that the specific anatomical variability of the cochlea of the patient plays an important role in the optimal insertion angle and depth. But the traditional Computerized Tomography (CT) or Cone Beam CT (CBCT) acquired prior to the surgery procedure cannot provide the surgeon with sufficient shape information given that the resolution of the current devices is not high enough to capture the small structures of the cochlea.

In this paper we present a software for planning electrode array insertion, that enriches conventional imaging based planning with data coming from high resolution models adapted to the patient specific anatomy. The rest of the paper is organized as follows: Sect. 2 describes the overall infrastructure of the software. Section 3 describes the modules and methods used by the application. Section 4 includes final remarks and future work.

2   Software Description

The outcome of the surgical procedure depends among other factors on the correct position of the CI's electrode array inside the cochlea and the depth of the insertion. However, conventional preoperative CT does not provide enough resolution to perform detailed analysis or simulations. High resolution models are needed to better evaluate the outcome of the procedure. The application presented herein is designed to provide surgeons with insight of what happens inside the cochlea when the electrode is inserted.

By combining high resolution models with patient-specific information, we can use several analysis tools that would be difficult to use with the low resolution pre-clinical data. Out application closes the gap between the clinical planning stage and advanced high resolution tools applied to the electrode insertion stage. This is achieved following a workflow (Fig. 2) of tasks that starts with the patient's pre-clinical images and ends with cochlea response simulations after the implantation procedure.

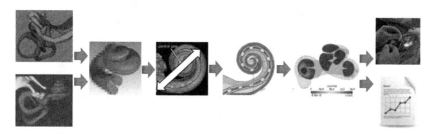

Fig. 2. Workflow of the software. From left to right: segmented structures and high resolution Statistical Shape Model as input. Patient-specific high resolution fitting. Cochlea Characterization, virtual insertion, electrical simulation, and finally, surgery and reporting.

The software runs on top of solid proven open source technologies as shown in Fig. 3. It is designed to be agnostic of operating system so it is compatible with the most popular operating systems. The Visualization Toolkit (VTK) is used as main graphical library. Qt and the Common Toolkit (CTK) are the basis of the User Interface. The communication with the clinical planning software [5] is performed using XML files defining the CT/CBCT and the segmented structures, as well as the planned path, safety volumes and any other patient relevant data.

3   Modular Structure

The software is comprised of different modules (Fig. 3) that provide individual information: patient specific high resolution anatomy model, cochlear characterization, virtual electrode insertion, electrical simulation and reporting.

3.1   Patient Specific Anatomy Model

To improve visualization and allow a more detailed modeling, a Statistical Shape Model (SSM) has been built using 17 microCT (μCT) samples of cadaveric temporal bone [7] obtained with Scanco Medical AG microCT-100 at 24 micron resolution. The inner ear structures were segmented semi-automatically using

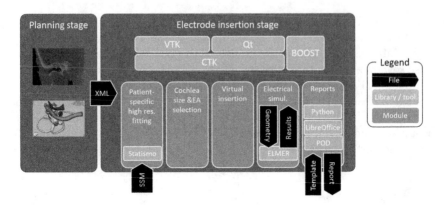

Fig. 3. Overview of the application structure, showing its modular structure as well as its software elements.

ITK-SNAP [13] and Seg3D2 [2]. The mesh resulting of the segmentations were post-processed using Markov Random Field Surface Reconstruction [10]. The datasets were registered (using Elastix [8]) to a image chosen as a reference. The transformation was applied to the reference segmentation so obtain the individual datasets with point correspondence. The SSM was built using the Statismo [9] software package. An Active Shape Model (ASM) is used to fit the high resolution model to the pre-clinical CT. The software allows inspection and generation of the SSM space through generation of specific samples (Fig. 4).

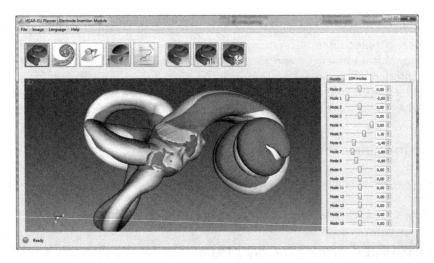

Fig. 4. Cochlear SSM loaded in the software. The mean shape of the SSM is displayed in white. Patient specific models can be generated according to the low resolution anatomy.

3.2   Cochlear Characterization

Measuring the cochlear size and shape is the first step to a correct electrode implant. The length of the cochlear duct, and the patient specific hearing impairment are key information to select the best fitting EA. The length of the unrolled cochlea has been extensively studied, and literature reports a 40 % variability with cochlear length ranging from 25 to 36 mm [6]. The final maximum insertion depth of the cochlear implant EA correlates with the diameter of the cochlea in the basal turn plane measured from the round window to the distal lateral wall [3]. This, in turn, enables the selection of the ideal electrode array from the portfolio of electrode array types that are integrated in the application (Fig. 5).

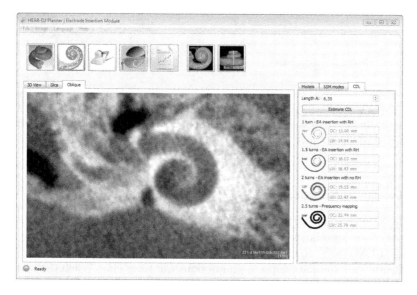

Fig. 5. Using the measurement from the diameter of the cochlea at the basal turn, the application estimates the unrolled length of the cochlea, and the different insertion depths of the electrode array.

3.3   Virtual Insertion

Once we have the patient's specific shape and a suitable electrode array has been selected, we can simulate the expected activation patterns of the implant. The last element needed for the simulation is to set the (virtual) position of the electrode array inside of the scala tympani, the chamber of the cochlea where the electrode is placed. An iterative method is used to compute the trajectory of a free-fitting electrode array, given the insertion point and direction. At each iteration the position and direction of the electrode tip with respect to the scala tympani is evaluated, ensuring that the tip proceeds tangentially and its distance from the wall is at least equal to the array radius. At each step the angle of impact to the wall and the margin between the cochlear implant array and the cochlear walls are evaluated too, providing an indirect measure of pressure against the wall. The iteration can stop prematurely if the electrode does not fit in the scala tympani dimensions or if it is subjected to excessive bending (Fig. 6).

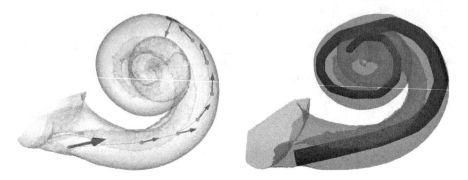

Fig. 6. Virtual insertion. Left: At each step of the insertion simulation, the tip position respect to the wall is evaluated and the direction is adjusted in order to lie tangentially to the wall. Right: Simulated electrode insertion. The final trajectory of the electrode is tangential to the scala tympani wall.

3.4   Electrical Simulations

The placed electrode is the last required step to perform the electrode simulations [1]. The simulation is performed using the multiphysics Finite Element Method (FEM) open source solver software ELMER [11]. In its current stage, the software can simulate bipolar simulation protocols (Fig. 7, left), where one electrode emits electrical current and the other is set to ground. Simulations also include modelizations of the electrical properties of nerve the fibers that start at the organ of Corti in the basilar membrane and form the auditory nerve, using the Generalized Schwarz-Eikhof-Frijns (GSEF) model [4] (Fig. 7, right).

3.5   Reporting

During the planning process, the operator has the option to save screenshots, possibly annotated with relevant information. After the process, the commented screenshots, along with the patient's clinical data, a Portable Document Format (PDF) report is generated for clinicians to review. The generation of the report employs the open source LibreOffice engine and POD (Python Open Document)[1] library to generate the report. For the generation of the reports with these technologies, a series of document templates are created that include embedded

---

[1] http://appyframework.org/pod.html.

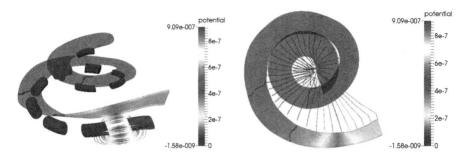

Fig. 7. Visualization of the simulation results. The basilar membrane has been rendered semitransparent for ease of visualization. Left: bipolar stimulation protocol of first two electrodes. Right: Nerve fiber stimulation after electrode activation pattern

Python code inserted into the document structure. The templates are post-processed using a Python script that can execute the embedded Python code and perform the adequate substitution of the variables. These variables include patient information and user generated screenshots and captions (Fig. 8).

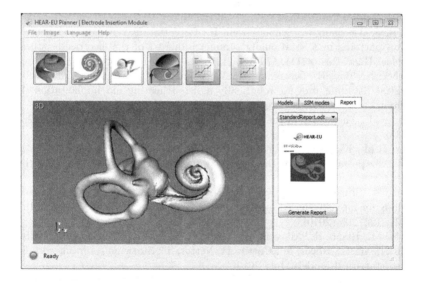

Fig. 8. Report generation interface.

4 Conclusions and Future Work

We have presented a software for the estimation of the patient specific inner ear and intra-cochlear anatomy, the planning and simulation of both the electrode insertion procedure, and the outcome of the surgery to the hearing capabilities for the patient. The software represents also a tool for the selection of the best electrode array for the patient and the reporting of the surgical procedure, making it a helping tool in the clinical practice. While the software is still evolving, it represents a collaborative effort in integrating many medical imaging tools, bringing the pre-surgery planning to a new level of information analysis.

Future work includes additional integration with more electrode models and tools from the electrode manufacturer, improvements on the virtual insertion phase using real-time simulation, and validation of the electrical simulations using audiometric tests are some of the future tasks planned for the software.

References

1. Ceresa, M., Mangado, N., Dejea, H., Carranza, N., Mistrik, P., Kjer, H.M., Vera, S., Paulsen, R., Ballester, M.A.: Patient-specific simulation of implant placement and function for cochlear implantation surgery planning (2014)
2. CIBC, Seg3D: Volumetric Image Segmentation and Visualization. Scientific Computing and Imaging Institute (SCI) (2014). http://www.seg3d.org
3. Escudé, B., James, C., Deguine, O., Cochard, N., Eter, E., Fraysse, B.: The size of the cochlea and predictions of insertion depth angles for cochlear implant electrodes. Audiol. Neurotol. **11**(1), 27–33 (2006)
4. Frijns, J., De Snoo, S., Schoonhoven, R.: Potential distributions and neural excitation patterns in a rotationally symmetric model of the electrically stimulated cochlea. Hear. Res. **87**(1), 170–186 (1995)
5. Gerber, N., Bell, B., Gavaghan, K., Weisstanner, C., Caversaccio, M., Weber, S.: Surgical planning tool for robotically assisted hearing aid implantation. Int. J. Comput. Assist. Radiol. Surg. **9**, 11–20 (2014)
6. Hardy, M.: The length of the organ of Corti in man. Am. J. Anat. **62**(2), 291–311 (1938)
7. Kjer, H.M., Fagertun, J., Vera, S., Pérez, F., González-Ballester, M.A., Paulsen, R.R.: Shape modelling of the inner ear from micro-CT data. In: SHAPE 2014 (2014)
8. Klein, S., Staring, M., Murphy, K., Viergever, M.A., Pluim, J.P.W.: elastix: A toolbox for intensity-based medical image registration. IEEE Trans. Med. Imaging **29**(1), 196–205 (2010)
9. Lüthi, M., Blanc, R., Albrecht, T., Gass, T., Goksel, O., Büchler, P., Kistler, M., Bousleiman, H., Reyes, M., Cattin, P., Vetter, T.: Statismo - a framework for pca based statistical models, July 2012
10. Paulsen, R., Bærentzen, J., Larsen, R.: Markov random field surface reconstruction. IEEE Trans. Vis. Comput. Graph. **16**(4), 636–646 (2010)
11. Ruokolainen, J., Lyly, M.: ELMER, a computational tool for PDEs-Application to vibroacoustics. CSC News **12**(4), 30–32 (2000)
12. World Health Organization. Deafness and hearing impairment (2012)
13. Yushkevich, P., Piven, J., Cody, H., Ho, S., Gee, J.C., Gerig, G.: User-guided level set segmentation of anatomical structures with ITK-SNAP. NeuroImage **31**, 1116–1128 (2005)

Weighted Partitioned Active Shape Model for Optic Pathway Segmentation in MRI

Xue Yang[1], Juan Cerrolaza[1], Chunzhe Duan[1], Qian Zhao[1],
Jonathan Murnick[2], Nabile Safdar[1,2], Robert Avery[3],
and Marius George Linguraru[1,4(✉)]

[1] Sheikh Zayed Institute for Pediatric Surgical Innovation,
Children's National Health System, Washington, DC, USA
[2] Division of Diagnostic Imaging and Radiology,
Children's National Health System, Washington, DC, USA
[3] Neurofibromatosis Institute, Children's National Health System,
Washington, DC, USA
[4] Departments of Radiology and Pediatrics, School of Medicine and Health
Sciences, George Washington University, Washington, DC, USA
mlingura@cnmc.org

Abstract. Active shape models (ASMs) have been established as robust model-based segmentation approaches and have been particularly relevant for objects ill-defined in image data. For example, the automatic segmentation of the optic pathway is almost impossible without shape models due to low contrast in MRI and local anatomical variability. However, traditional ASM is not optimal for complex or variable shapes segmentation due to its strong constraints. Herein, we introduce a weighted partitioned active shape model to improve the shape flexibility and robustness of ASMs and apply it to optic pathway (including the nerve, chiasm, and tract) segmentation. The strong constraints of ASM are relaxed by partitioning the whole shape into several subparts. In this way, the local shape variability can be captured and the number of training data can be reduced. Our novel weighted matching approach assigns a weight to each landmark point according to its appearance confidence, thus deforming the shape to reliable positions. In the application of optic pathway segmentation, the mean of root mean squared symmetric surface distance is 0.59 mm, which is about one voxel size.

Keywords: Optic pathway segmentation · Active shape model · Partitioned ASM · Weighted ASM · MRI

1 Introduction

Statistical shape models (SSMs) have been widely applied in medical image segmentations and been established as robust model-based segmentation approaches [1]. Active shape models (ASMs) [2] are some of the best-known SSMs gathering the information about mean shape and common variations through statistical training. However, traditional ASMs are often over-constrained and insufficient training data can lead to considerable errors [3]. In recent years, many efforts have been contributed to increase shape model flexibility. De Bruijne et al. [4] proposed a flexible shape model

© Springer International Publishing Switzerland 2014
M.G. Linguraru et al. (Eds.): CLIP 2014, LNCS 8680, pp. 109–117, 2014.
DOI: 10.1007/978-3-319-13909-8_14

for tubular structure segmentation by modeling axis and cross-sectional shape deformation separately. This approach was demonstrated to increase the flexibility of the
shape model and work well in abdominal aortic aneurysms segmentation, but it
requires the image slices to be approximately perpendicular to the object axis which is
hard to ensure in many other applications. Zhao et al. [5] proposed a partitioned ASM
for brain MRI segmentation by automatically partitioning the faces of a mesh into a
group of tiles. They proved their model outperformed traditional ASM and Hierarchical
ASM [6] in some brain structure segmentations. However, their partitioning method
randomly selected a face in each tile growing may miss some anatomic structural
information and the partitioned results may vary on each run.

Morphological assessments of the optic pathway and its lesions are important in the
assessment, diagnosis and monitoring of many vision-threatening conditions. These
conditions may be demonstrated on imaging by a decrease in the size of the optic
nerve, chiasm and tracts. On the other hand, optic pathway gliomas (OPGs), the most
frequently identified brain tumor in children with neurofibromatosis type 1 (NF1) [7],
may increase the size of these structures and require an accurate quantitative measurement of tumor growth to provide effective management and assessment of therapeutic response. However, traditional measurements of structures, like bi-dimensional
diameter product are often imprecise and irreproducible [8]. To allow accurate morphological analysis, we propose an automatic method to segment the optic pathway.

Automatic segmentation of optic pathway is challenging because of the thin and
long structure and low contrast in MRI; little work has been previously proposed in this
area. Bekes et al. [9] proposed a geometrical model for eyeballs, lenses, and optic
nerves segmentation, but the reproducibility of optic nerves and chiasms may below
50 %. Noble [10] proposed a medial axis and deformable model with level-set method
to segment optic nerves and chiasm using MR and CT images. They reported good
performance on optic nerves and chiasm, but they did not include optic tracts, which
are the most challenging to segment.

The optic pathway has globally well-defined shape, but locally variable. To address
its automatic segmentation, we introduce a weighted partitioned active shape model
(WP-ASM). Our main contributions are: (1) proposal of a new hierarchical partitioned
ASM; (2) definition of an appearance-based weight matrix with application of weighted
matching in the partitioned model framework; (3) adaptation of an automatic landmark
clustering in the use of partitioned ASM; (4) combination of intensity and tubular
structure features in the appearance model; (5) application of our WP-ASM to whole
optic pathway (including nerves, chiasm and tracts) segmentation in T1 weighted MRI.
The partitioned model provides flexible shape modeling and the weighted matching
method improves the robustness of deformable shapes. Our methodology is general and
its robustness to the segmentation of the optic pathway shows its applicability to the
analysis of objects with complex and variable shapes in image data.

2   Methods

In traditional ASMs [2], landmark points are used to describe object shape and shape
variations using point distribution model (PDM). The landmark points on each training

example are represented by a shape vector and aligned to a common coordinate system. Principle Component Analysis (PCA) is applied to the aligned shape vectors to generate the shape model.

$$x = \bar{x} + \Phi b \tag{1}$$

where x represents an aligned training shape vector, $\bar{x}$ is the mean shape vector, Φ consists eigenvectors corresponding to selected largest eigenvalues, and b is a vector of shape parameters for each mode. For a given shape vector x, the shape parameter vector b is calculated as

$$b = \Phi^{\top}(x - \bar{x}) \tag{2}$$

To constrain the generated shape similar to the learning shape during training, b is limited to a certain interval.

2.1   Partitioned ASM

To capture local variations during shape learning, we automatically partition the whole surface into subparts based on a clustering process, which captures the anatomical variability of single shape via principal component or factor analysis [11]. Here we use a more general approach based on the agglomerative hierarchical clustering method presented by Ward [12]. In this automatic partition method, the user can define the number of partitions. Optic pathway is a tubular structure and it is desirable to maintain this tubular property in subparts. We performed experiments for different numbers of partitions and chose the configuration producing almost small tube-like structures. Experimentally, we chose 16 partitions.

To ensure that adjacent partitions are connected during model fitting, we introduce overlapping areas between partitions. After automatic partition, the landmark points are divided into disconnect partitions (i.e., one landmark point can only be in one partition). Thus, some faces of the whole surface are removed. To get overlapping partitions, we add landmark points connected by these removed faces to each partition. Then some points, which are referred to as joint points, will appear in more than one partition. During model fitting, we calculate the shape parameters for each partition separately, and then the shape parameters of the joint points are computed as the mean shape parameters from their partitions. By introducing joint points, the connections of partitions are maintained. The results of 16 overlapping partitions are shown in Fig. 1 with the first mode of variation for five example partitions.

In traditional ASM, after applying PCA, each training example is represented by the shape parameters in a hyperspace defined by eigenvectors. In partitioned ASM, if we combine the partitioned H hyperspaces to one hyperspace, each training example can be represented by a curve in the new hyperspace as proposed by Zhao [5]. Zhao el al. aligned the test model curve to its closest training curve during model fitting to keep the shape plausible. However, it is possible that the curve of a plausible shape is not similar to any training curve. To relax this assumption, we propose a hierarchical shape model by fitting a second level PCA to the curve in the new hyperspace. Compared to Eq. (1), we have

$$x_h = \overline{x_h} + \Phi_h b_h,$$
(3)

$$z = \bar{z} + P\beta,$$
(4)

where h indicates the index of the partition, x_h is a shape vector for partition h, $z = [\, b_1 \quad b_2 \quad \cdots \quad b_H \,]^\top$ is a vector combining all shape parameters representing the corresponding curve in the hyperspace, and P consists eigenvectors of the curve in the hyperspace. The value of β can be constrained to ensure that the deformable shape will not be far from the training shape. During model fitting, the value of the landmark position x_h is updated in every iteration using Eq. (3) to exclude noise, while the value of z is updated only if it falls out of the constrained range.

2.2   Appearance Model

The optic pathway is a thin and long structure surrounded by a variety of types of tissues with variable appearance. When the optic pathway is closed to brain structures the contrast to noise level is low and makes the segmentation difficult. Therefore, the traditional local appearance model using normalized derivatives along a profile [13] is not robust. To adapt the local appearance model to thin structure segmentation, we define a sub-voxel step size between voxels in a profile. We apply a three-class fuzzy c-means filter and use the second class probability as the tissue intensity probability to distinguish the optic pathway from the surrounding darker or brighter structures. Besides, the tubular structure of the optic pathway is enhanced using the spherical flux [14] as another feature in the appearance model.

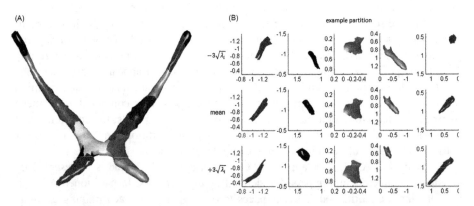

Fig. 1. Automatic Partition Results. (A) is the colored surface of the optic pathway showing the results of the automatic 16 partitions where different colors represent different partitions. (B) shows the first mode of variation for five partitions color-matched with (A). The first two columns are two partitions in left and right optic nerves, the middle column is a partition in optic chiasm, and the last two columns are two partitions in left and right optic tracts (Colour figure online).

Finally, the normalized derivatives, the tissue intensity probabilities, and the tubular structure probabilities are used together to train the local structure for each landmark point. For each landmark profile, the interpolations of these three feature images are put in a single vector, and the mean value and covariance of this vector are calculated across training examples. This combination is designed to increase the robustness of the appearance model to variable image environment. The optimal position for each landmark point is computed by minimizing the Mahalanobis distance [13].

2.3   Weighted Shape Matching

The optic pathway can be easily distinguished from surrounding tissues in some places (in fatty areas) while harder in others (inside the gray matter). Thus, in finding the best nearby point based on the appearance cost function, we have different confidence levels for different landmark points. Using this confidence value, we can estimate weighted shape parameters that attract the points to reliable positions. As proposed in [15], the weighted shape parameter for each partition is computed as

$$ b_h = \left(\Phi_h^\top W_h \Phi_h \right)^{-1} \Phi_h^\top W_h (x_h - \overline{x_h}), \tag{5} $$

where W_h is a diagonal weight matrix for partition h with corresponding weight value for each landmark.

We assume that if the variance of the appearance profile is low, the confidence we have on this landmark point is high. Thus, the weight of a landmark is proportional to the inverse value of the profile variance. We define the weight for landmark point i as

$$ w_i = \frac{1}{(1 + \mathrm{tr}(S_i))}, \tag{6} $$

where S_i is the covariance matrix of the appearance model for landmark point i, and $\mathrm{tr}(S_i)$ represents the trace of the matrix, which is the total variance of the profile.

3   Experiments and Results

Seventeen MRIs of children with healthy optic pathways were acquired for this study. The children were aged from 1 year old to 17 years old. The MRIs were T1 weighted cube with contrast enhancement (Gd) with resolutions from $0.39 \times 0.60 \times 0.39$ mm^3 to $0.47 \times 0.60 \times 0.47$ mm^3. The optic pathways in MR images were manually segmented by either an expert neuro-radiologist or an expert neuro-ophthalmologist for gold standard.

One dataset was selected as the reference set, the left datasets were divided into training set and testing set; we used a leave-one-out cross-validation to evaluate our model performance. During training, all the training images were registered to the reference set using affine registration implemented in NiftyReg [16]. The twelve registration parameters were first optimized for the whole brain, and then further optimized over the region of interest containing the optic pathway, which was manually identified.

After registration, the surfaces for each training example were calculated using methods proposed in [17]. The landmark points were defined by non-linearly registering the reference surface to every other training surface using point set registration [18] and IRTK toolbox [19]. The shape model was learned for each partition after removing the translations, rotations and scales of the whole optic pathway. The appearance model for each landmark was learned by sampling along the landmark normal direction 5 voxels on each side with 0.25 voxel distance. The normalized derivative, the tissue intensity probability, and the tubular structure probability from the spherical flux response were used together to learn appearance model, which resulted in 33 elements in each appearance vector.

During testing, the test set was registered to the reference set using affine registration. Then the WP-ASM was performed on the affine registered image. The mean shape of the training set was used as the initial surface for ASM segmentation. The landmark points were optimized from a rough to fine image scale (0.25, 0.5 and 1).

To evaluate the segmentation performance, the Dice similarity coefficient (DSC), the symmetric mean surface distance (MSD), the symmetric root mean squared points-to-surface error (RMSE), and the relative volume error (RVE) were calculated for each leave-one-out test. The symmetric MSD and RMSE were computed as the mean of both directions of distance from the expert labels to the estimated segmentations and vice versa. The relative volume error was computed as the volume error proportional to the volume of the ground truth. Quantitative results are shown in Fig. 2 and Table 1. Qualitative results of the worst case (maximum RMSE) and the best case (minimum RMSE) are displayed in Fig. 3. The results of our proposed method were compared with traditional ASM. The traditional ASM used the whole shape for shape model training and the normalized derivative for appearance model while other parameters were the same. The difference between our WP-ASM and traditional ASM were tested using Wilcoxon signed rank test. WP-ASM performed significantly better than ASM on all metrics. On average, WP-ASM estimated the size of the long and thin optic pathway with 10 % RVE versus 77 % RVE for ASM.

4   Discussion

ASMs struggle to segment complex, irregular objects in image data. In this paper, we introduced a new WP-ASM approach and applied it to the segmentation of the optic

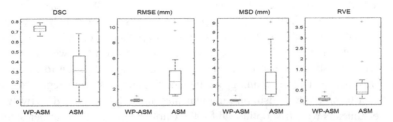

Fig. 2. Quantitative results comparing our proposed weighted partitioned ASM (WP-ASM) with original ASM.

Table 1. Sumary of segmentation results.

	DSC	RMSE (mm)	MSD (mm)	RVE
ASM	0.31 ± 0.19	3.66 ± 2.89	2.82 ± 2.35	0.77 ± 0.91
WP-ASM	0.73 ± 0.04	0.59 ± 0.17	0.44 ± 0.14	0.10 ± 0.10
Wilcoxon test	p = 4.4e−4	p = 4.4e−4	p = 4.4e−4	p = 0.001

pathway (including the nerve, chiasm, and tract). The partitioned shape model provides more flexibility for shape evolution, and the weighted matching method makes the deformable shape more reliable. We used an automatic partitioning of the model based on clustering, and overlaying areas between partitions to ensure connectivity. An appearance model adaptable to variable image environment was also embedded to increase the robustness of the segmentation.

The general segmentation method that we proposed was applied to the automatic optic pathway segmentation in T1 MRI image. The mean of the RMSE across 16 test sets was 0.59 mm, which is about 1 voxel size. The DSC is smaller than the method proposed in [10], but their method required matched CT and MRI images, which is not part of the pediatric clinical protocol and involves radiation. Besides, we segmented the whole optic pathway (including the tract) while other segmentation approaches only work on optic nerves and chiasm segmentation.

Since the optic pathway is a very thin structure the average DSC is unsurprisingly not high. From Fig. 2 we can see that the hardest part of the optic pathway segmentation is the optic tract. To more accurately evaluate our results we will compare the performance to inter-rater similarity in future work. At this stage, we do not have data for inter-rater evaluation, but this will be address in the future.

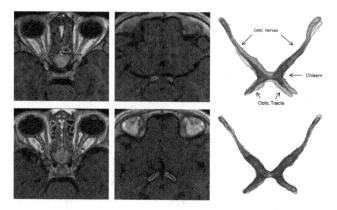

Fig. 3. Automatic Segmentation Results. The first row shows the worst case of automatic segmentation results (RMSE = 1.14 mm) and the second row shows the best case (RMSE = 0.43 mm). In green we show the manual label and in red is the automatic segmentation. The left column shows and axial image of the optic nerves, the middle column shows the optic tracts, and the right column displays the overlaid manual and automatic segmentation surfaces (Colour figure online).

Our automatic segmentation outperforms most previously presented work for localizing these structures [9]. An additional advantage is that our WP-ASM lowers the degrees of freedom in shape training and requires less training examples to build an accurate shape model. Automated segmentation of the optic pathways using these methods could serve a useful function in the more precise evaluation of conditions affecting these structures like optic nerve glioma. Because of the local flexibility, our proposed WP-ASM may be adapted to segment optic path gliomas and other complex and irregular structures in image data.

Acknowledgements. This project was supported in part by the Neurofibromatosis Institute at Children's National and a philanthropic gift from the Government of Abu Dhabi to Children's National Healthcare System.

References

1. Heimann, T., et al.: Statistical shape models for 3D medical image segmentation: a review. Med. Image Anal. **13**, 543–563 (2009)
2. Cootes, T.F., et al.: Active shape models-their training and application. Comput. Vis. Image Underst. **61**, 38–59 (1995)
3. Lamecker, H., et al.: Segmentation of the liver using a 3D statistical shape model. Citeseer, Kyoto (2004)
4. de Bruijne, M., et al.: Adapting active shape models for 3D segmentation of tubular structures in medical images. Inf. Process. Med. Imaging **18**, 136–147 (2003)
5. Zhao, Z., et al.: A novel 3D partitioned active shape model for segmentation of brain MR images. Med. Image Comput. Comput.-Assist. Interv. **3749**, 221–228 (2005)
6. Davatzikos, C., et al.: Hierarchical active shape models, using the wavelet transform. IEEE Trans. Med. Imaging **22**, 414–423 (2003)
7. Avery, R.A., et al.: Optic pathway gliomas. J. Neuroophthalmol. Off. J. North Am. Neuroophthalmol. Soc. **31**, 269–278 (2011)
8. Schmitt, P., et al.: Effects of slice thickness and head rotation when measuring glioma sizes on MRI: in support of volume segmentation versus two largest diameters methods. J. Neurooncol. **112**, 165–172 (2013)
9. Bekes, G., et al.: Geometrical model-based segmentation of the organs of sight on CT images. Med. Phys. **35**, 735–743 (2008)
10. Noble, J.H., et al.: An atlas-navigated optimal medial axis and deformable model algorithm (NOMAD) for the segmentation of the optic nerves and chiasm in MR and CT images. Med. Image Anal. **15**, 877–884 (2011)
11. Reyes, M., et al.: Anatomical variability of organs via principal factor analysis from the construction of an abdominal probabilistic atlas. In: Proceedings IEEE International Symposium on Biomedical Imaging, vol. 2009, pp. 682–685 (2009)
12. Ward Jr., J.H.: Hierarchical grouping to optimize an objective function. J. Am. Stat. Assoc. **58**, 236–244 (1963)
13. Cootes, T.F., et al.: Statistical models of appearance for medical image analysis and computer vision. In: SPIE Medical Imaging, pp. 236–248 (2001)
14. Law, M.W., et al.: Efficient implementation for spherical flux computation and its application to vascular segmentation. IEEE Trans. Image Process. Publ. IEEE Signal Process. Soc. **18**, 596–612 (2009)

15. Zhao, M., et al.: Shape evaluation for weighted active shape models. In: Proceedings of the Asian Conference on Computer Vision, pp. 1074–1079 (2004)
16. Ourselin, S., et al.: Robust registration of multi-modal images: towards real-time clinical applications. In: Dohi, T., Kikinis, R. (eds.) MICCAI 2002, Part II. LNCS, vol. 2489. Springer, Heidelberg (2002)
17. Fang, Q., et al.: Tetrahedral mesh generation from volumetric binary and grayscale images. In: ISBI'09. IEEE International Symposium on, pp. 1142–1145 (2009)
18. Myronenko, A., et al.: Point set registration: coherent point drift. IEEE Trans. Pattern Anal. Mach. Intell. **32**, 2262–2275 (2010)
19. Rueckert, D., et al.: Nonrigid registration using free-form deformations: application to breast MR images. IEEE Trans. Med. Imaging **18**, 712–721 (1999)

Longitudinal Intensity Normalization in Multiple Sclerosis Patients

Yogesh Karpate$^{(\boxtimes)}$, Olivier Commowick, Christian Barillot, and Gilles Edan

VISAGES: INSERM U746 - CNRS UMR6074 - INRIA - University of Rennes I,
Rennes, France
Yogesh.Karpate@irisa.fr

Abstract. In recent years, there have been many Multiple Sclerosis (MS) studies using longitudinal MR images to study and characterize the MS lesion patterns. The intensity of similar anatomical tissues in MR images is often different because of the variability of the acquisition process and different scanners. This paper proposes a novel methodology for a longitudinal lesion analysis based on intensity standardization to minimize the inter-scan intensity difference. The intensity normalization maps parameters obtained using a robust Gaussian Mixture Model (GMM) estimation not affected by the presence of MS lesions. Experimental results demonstrate that our technique accurately performs the task of intensity standardization. We show consequently how the same technique can improve the results of longitudinal MS lesion detection.

1 Introduction

Multiple Sclerosis (MS) is an acquired inflammatory, demyelinating disease which causes disabilities in young adults and it is very common in the northern hemisphere. Quantitative analysis of longitudinal Magnetic Resonance Images (MRI) of subject taken at different time points provides a time varying analysis of the brain tissues which may lead to the discovery of new biomarkers of disease evolution. In MS, White Matter (WM) lesions are also present in addition to healthy brain tissues. Lesions can remain stationary, change volume, or disappear in later time points depending upon the state of MS. Due to protocol variations in the scanners, following the evolution of tissue intensities in a patient, e.g. changing appearance of lesions, makes quantitative evaluation of lesions difficult. In order to alleviate this problem, intensity normalization is necessary.

Histogram matching is a widely used technique in intensity standardization. In their seminal work, Nyul et al. [7] proposed landmark based methods. It consists of matching the input image histogram landmarks onto standard histogram landmarks, obtained in a training phase, performing a linear interpolation of intensities between the positions. The technique in [7] uses percentile landmarks, which is simple yet powerful. Jager et al. [5] extended this principle to two or more jointly used MRI sequences (e.g., T1-w and T2-w), matching multidimensional joint histograms with nonlinear registration. With this method, no prior registration of the reference and normalized MR images is required.

© Springer International Publishing Switzerland 2014
M.G. Linguraru et al. (Eds.): CLIP 2014, LNCS 8680, pp. 118–125, 2014.
DOI: 10.1007/978-3-319-13909-8_15

An algorithm proposed by Wang et al. [12] expands or shrinks a windowed part of the input image histogram with a multiplicative factor, found by minimizing the bin-count difference between the source and moving images histograms. The window is used to include only voxels of interest and exclude the background. This makes the technique linear in the intensity range of interest. Other techniques use parametric models, such as the technique proposed by Hellier [4]. It models histogram of a reference image and of the standardized image with two GMMs and aligns their means through a polynomial correction function. Weisenfeld et.al. [13] have proposed to estimate a multiplicative correction field that alters the intensity statistics of an image or set of images to best match those of a model. In that paper, the Kullback-Leibler divergence between the source and moving images is minimized iteratively to estimate the parameters of a model, thus histograms are equalized. All these methods may be affected by the presence of white matter lesions.

We propose a longitudinal intensity normalization algorithm for multichannel MRI in the presence of MS lesions, which provides consistent and reliable longitudinal detections. The tissue intensities from multichannel MRI are modeled with parametric transform using a robust GMM estimation based on γ divergence, thereby keeping the lesions unaffected. The proposed technique is built on ideas similar to Hellier [4] but taking into account the presence of pathological tissues in the intensity transformation function. It provides a technique that (1) uses tissue-specific intensity information by modeling them using a robust GMM; (2) provides a consistent intensity normalization between longitudinal images. Subsequently, we demonstrate its crucial role for further lesion analysis.

This paper is organized as follows. The modeling and parameter estimation of multi-sequence MRI with γ divergence followed by intensity normalization are reviewed in Sect. 2. The details of experiments and their results on longitudinal MS patients are discussed in Sect. 3.

2   Methodology

Given two MR images of a single MS patient at time instant t_1 and t_2, we seek to estimate a correction factor such that corresponding anatomical tissues adopt the same intensity profile. We model the image intensities of a healthy brain with a 3-class GMM, where each Gaussian represents one of the brain tissues White Matter (WM), Gray Matter(GM) and Cerebrospinal fluid (CSF). We consider the m MR sequences as a multidimensional image with n voxels. Each voxel i is represented as $\mathbf{x}_i = [x_{i1}...x_{im}]$. The probability of intensity $\mathbf{x}_i$ is calculated as follows:

$$f(\mathbf{x}_i|\theta) = \sum_{k=1}^{3} \pi_k \mathcal{N}(\mu_k, \Sigma_k) \tag{1}$$

where the mean μ_k and covariance Σ_k define the parameters $\mathcal{N}(\mu_k, \Sigma_k)$ of each Gaussian of the model along with their mixing proportions π_k merged into parameter θ. If the proportions were known, θ could be estimated through the Maximum Likelihood Estimator (MLE):

$$\hat{\theta} = \underset{\theta}{\text{argmax}}\ L(\theta) = \underset{\theta}{\text{argmax}} \prod_{i=1}^{n} f(\mathbf{x}_i|\theta) \tag{2}$$

Where $\mathbf{x}_i$ are considered as i.i.d. samples. However, as π_k are unknown, an Expectation Maximization (EM) algorithm [3] is used to estimate the parameters.

2.1 γ-loss Function for the Normal Distribution

The parameter estimation with classic MLE for GMM can deviate from its true estimation in presence of outliers. In MS patients, such outliers may be of crucial importance as they may denote appearing or disappearing lesions. Notsu et al. [6] proposed a modification of the MLE in order to make it more robust to outliers. The basic idea is to maximize (2) in the form of γ divergence. We consider the γ-loss function for the Normal distribution with mean vector μ and covariance matrix Σ.

$$L_\gamma(\mu, \Sigma) = \left|\Sigma^{-\frac{\gamma}{2(1+\gamma)}}\right| \sum_{i=1}^{n} \exp\left(-\frac{\gamma}{2}(\mathbf{x}_i - \mu)^T \Sigma^{-1}(\mathbf{x}_i - \mu)\right) \tag{3}$$

Where $|.|$ indicates the determinant. The bounded influence function of an estimator is an indicator of robustness to outliers. The influence function for GMM with γ loss function is bounded whereas the one for regular GMM is unbounded. As γ grows larger, bounds become tighter. For a sufficiently large γ, ($\gamma \geq 0.1$), the estimating equation has little impact from outliers contaminated in the data set. Equation (3) can be casted to yield an EM style algorithm as follows.

Expectation Step. In the case of a GMM, the latent variables are the point-to-cluster assignments $k_i, i = 1, ..., n$, one for each of n data points. The auxiliary distribution $q(k_i|\mathbf{x}_i) = q_{ik}$ is a matrix with $n \times K$ entries. Each row of q_i can be thought of as a vector of soft assignments of the data points $\mathbf{x}_i$ to each of the Gaussian modes.

$$q_{ik} = \frac{\pi_k \exp\left(-\frac{\gamma}{2}(\mathbf{x}_i - \mu_k)^T \Sigma_k^{-1}(\mathbf{x}_i - \mu_k)\right)}{\sum\limits_{l=1}^{K} \pi_l \exp\left(-\frac{\gamma}{2}(\mathbf{x}_i - \mu_l)^T \Sigma_l^{-1}(\mathbf{x}_i - \mu_l)\right)} \tag{4}$$

Maximization Step. The maximization step estimates the parameters of the Gaussian mixture components and the mixing proportions π_k, given the auxiliary distribution on the point-to-cluster assignments computed in the expectation step. The mean μ_k of a Gaussian mode is obtained as the mean of the data points assigned to it (accounting for the strength of the soft assignments). The other quantities are obtained in a similar manner, yielding to:

$$\mu_k = \frac{\sum_{i=1}^{n} q_{ik} \mathbf{x}_i}{\sum_{i=1}^{n} q_{ik}} \tag{5}$$

$$\Sigma_k = (1 + \gamma) \frac{\sum_{i=1}^{n} q_{ik} (\mathbf{x}_i - \mu_k)(\mathbf{x}_i - \mu_k)^T}{\sum_{i=1}^{n} q_{ik}} \tag{6}$$

$$\pi_k = \frac{\sum_{i=1}^{n} q_{ik}}{\sum_{i=1}^{n} \sum_{l=1}^{K} q_{il}} \tag{7}$$

2.2   Selection of Parameter γ

The estimation of power index γ plays a critical role in our approach, since γ affects the estimated parameters in presence of outliers. Notsu et al. [6] suggested the selection of γ as a model selection problem based on Akaike information criterion (AIC). Let K be the number of clusters, p be the total numbers of parameters of a model and (μ_k, Σ_k), $k = 1, .., K$ be the means and the covariance matrices of the clusters respectively. From (1), the AIC is defined as follows:

$$\mathbf{AIC}_\gamma = -2 \sum_{i=1}^{n} \log f_\gamma(\mathbf{x}_i | \theta) + 2 \left\{ K \frac{p(p+3)}{2} + K - 1 \right\} \tag{8}$$

The value of γ which minimizes AIC is used as the optimal γ. For various values of γ, Eq. (8) is evaluated in cross validation manner and the γ which results in minimum value is chosen for the experiment.

2.3   Intensity Correction

We obtain the means and covariances of tissues for the source and target images using the procedure mentioned above. We chose a linear correction function such that $g(\mathbf{x}) = \Sigma_i \beta_i \mathbf{x}_i$. The coefficients β_i are estimated to minimize the following cost function: $\Sigma_{l=1}^{l=n} (g(\mu_{source,k}) - \mu_{target,k})^2$. This function can be solved by linear regression. Using the results of the linear regression, the intensity profiles of the two images are normalized by mapping the intensity of the source image to the target image. The resulting correction function is smooth and interpolates the intensity correction.

3   Experiments and Results

3.1   Dataset and Preprocessing

Whole-brain MR images were acquired on 18 MS patients. T1-w MPRAGE, T2-w and FLAIR modalities were chosen for the experiment. Expert annotations of lesions were carried out by an expert radiologist on all MS patients. The volume size for T1-w MPRAGE and FLAIR is $256 \times 256 \times 160$ and voxel size is $1 \times 1 \times 1\,\mathrm{mm}^3$. For T2-w, the volume size is $256 \times 256 \times 44$ and voxel size is $1 \times 1 \times 3\,mm^3$. All imaging experiments for this study were performed on a 3T Siemens Verio (VB17) scanner with a 32-channel head coil. MR images from each patient are de-noised [2], bias field corrected [11] and registered with respect to T1-MPRAGE volume [1,9]. All the images are processed to extract intra-cranial region using **BET** (Brain Extraction Tool) [10].

We show the effect of longitudinal intensity normalization followed by detection on both normal tissues and lesions for 18 MS subjects, having 4 time-points each, approximately separated by a period of three to six months. The first time point is considered as the reference point to which the subsequent time points (moving ones) are aligned using intensity normalization. First, the parameters of reference and moving images are estimated using γ likelihood estimator as described in Sect. 2.1. Secondly, voxels of moving image are aligned with respect to reference image using the procedure in Sect. 2.3. Each patient and each time point $t = 2, ..., t_n$, are rigidly registered to the T1-w MPRAGE of first time instance. The obtained difference image is processed further to obtain a soft detection by using heuristic thresholding iteratively (1) by Otsu's threshold [8]; (2) erosion of image by one voxel. The detections from this difference image are compared with difference image of ground truth at corresponding time points.

3.2   Intensity Correction Evaluation

To evaluate the quality of intensity normalization, we compare the histograms of reference, moving and intensity normalized moving image using chi-squared distance given by $\chi^2_{x,y} = \frac{1}{2} \sum \frac{(x_i - y_i)^2}{x_i + y_i}$. Lower values of this distance indicate better alignment of intensities. Table 1 reports the chi-squared distance for various imaging sequences. Different methods are compared against the proposed one. We report the mean χ^2 distance for our method as 0.18($\pm$0.045), 0.28($\pm$0.037) 0.32($\pm$0.038) for T1-w MPRAGE, T2-w and FLAIR respectively, outperforming other state of the art methods.

Table 1. Chi-squared distance analysis for histogram matching

Modality	Before Normalization	After Normalization		
		Proposed	Hellier	Nyul
T1-w	0.56 ($\pm$0.03)	**0.18** ($\pm$0.045)	0.35 ($\pm$0.029)	0.3 ($\pm$0.019)
T2-w	0.62 ($\pm$0.029)	**0.28** ($\pm$0.037)	0.414 ($\pm$0.03)	0.315 ($\pm$0.042)
FLAIR	0.56 ($\pm$0.027)	**0.32** ($\pm$0.038)	0.45 ($\pm$0.051)	0.39 ($\pm$0.045)

Figure 1 shows the intensity correction results for T1-w MPRAGE, T2-w and FLAIR images. Three time points and their corresponding MR modalities of a subject are shown before and after normalization. Each row represents the imaging modality and each column depicts the first time point, second time point, the absolute difference image without and with intensity normalization respectively. This figure demonstrates visually the ability of our approach to

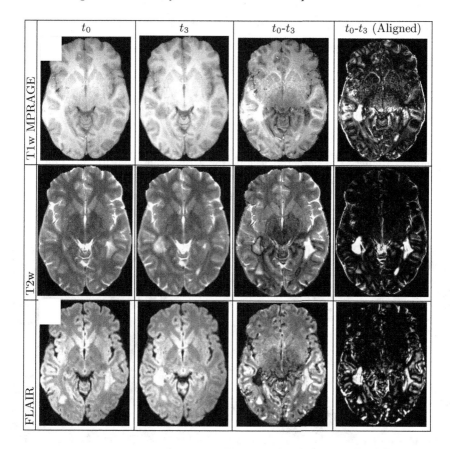

Fig. 1. Intensity correction

normalize intensities. As seen from the difference image of the first and second time points, intensity alignment reduces significantly the difference in intensities without affecting the lesion appearance. It will be easier to automatically detect evolving lesions on the images in the last column.

3.3   Longitudinal Lesion Detection

To show the quantitative improvement for identification of lesions, we report in Table 2 the precision (Positive Predicted Value) and recall (Sensitivity) of lesion detection averaged across the 18 patients for various overlap thresholds. The lesion is said to be detected if $\frac{R_c \cap R_{GT}}{R_{GT}} \geq \varphi$ where R_c, R_{GT} and φ are respectively the candidate region in the image, the ground truth and a threshold. Table 2 reports values of precision and recall for various thresholds. As from the figures, our approach outperforms other methods. We have a very high recall of 0.90 at $\varphi = 0.2$ and 0.82 even at $\varphi = 0.4$.

Table 2. Performance analysis for lesion detection.

Method	$\varphi = 0.2$		$\varphi = 0.3$		$\varphi = 0.4$	
	Precision	Recall	Precision	Recall	Precision	Recall
Nyul	0.63±0.01	0.60±0.02	0.61±0.04	0.67±0.02	0.58±0.03	0.64±0.03
Proposed	**0.73±0.04**	**0.90±0.05**	**0.68±0.03**	**0.85±0.04**	**0.63±0.03**	**0.82±0.01**
Hellier	0.65±0.02	0.74±0.03	0.64±0.06	0.68±0.04	0.62±0.03	0.59±0.05

Figure 2 depicts the detected lesions for a representative image. The green label shows new lesions at t_3, orange shows stationary lesions which are also a part of t_1; blue shows false positive detections. We are able to accurately detect appearing and disappearing lesions thanks to the proposed method.

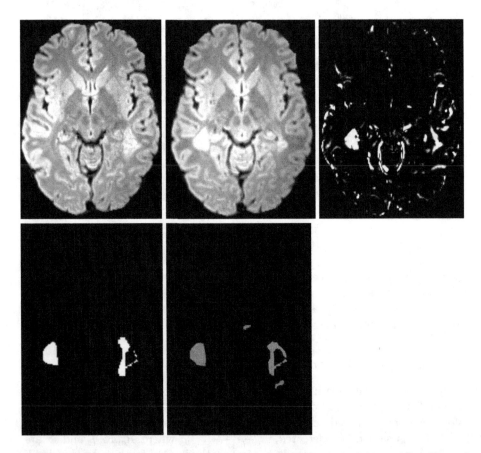

Fig. 2. Lesion detection examples. For top and bottom, from left to right: Slice of FLAIR for t_0, t_3, $|t_0 - t_{3(Normalized)}|$, ground truth and lesions detected by our algorithm (Color figure online).

4   Discussion and Conclusion

We proposed a new intensity normalization technique based on a robust GMM estimation with γ divergence. The efficacy of our method was evaluated through histogram matching distance method and longitudinal lesion detection. Compared to Nyul and Hellier method, our methodology is more suitable for longitudinal MS lesion analysis because of its ability to preserve the intensity variations caused by pathological changes. Our system relies heavily on a robust parametric modeling of tissue intensities based on γ divergence. The resulting system is both efficient and accurate, outperforming the state of the art methods. This performance suggests that it can provide valuable assistance in detecting the longitudinal MS lesions in clinical routine with high reliability. Our models are already capable of detecting highly variable lesion patterns, but we would like to move towards richer models. The framework described here allows for exploration of additional MR sequences with or without contrast agents. For example, one can consider infusing T1-w Gadolinium and DTI.

References

1. Commowick, O., Wiest-Daesslé, N., Prima, S.: Block-matching strategies for rigid registration of multimodal medical images. In: ISBI, pp. 700–703 (2012)
2. Coupé, P., Yger, P., Prima, S., Hellier, P., Kervrann, C., Barillot, C.: An optimized blockwise nonlocal means denoising filter for 3-D magnetic resonance images. IEEE TMI **27**(4), 425–441 (2008)
3. Dempster, A., Laird, N., Rubin, D.: Maximum likelihood from incomplete data via the EM algorithm. J. Roy. Stat. Soc.: Ser. B **39**(1), 1–38 (1977)
4. Hellier, P.: Consistent intensity correction of MR images. In: ICIP, pp. 1109–1112 (2003)
5. Jäger, F., Nyul, L., Frericks, B., Wacker, F., Hornegger, J.: Whole body MRI intensity standardization. In: Horsch, A., Deserno, T.M., Handels, H., Meinzer, H.-P., Tolxdorff, T. (eds.) Bildverarbeitung für die Medizin, pp. 459–463. Springer, Heidelberg (2007)
6. Notsu, A., Komori, O., Eguchi, S.: Spontaneous clustering via minimum gamma-divergence. Neural Comput. **26**(2), 421–448 (2014)
7. Nyul, L., Udupa, J., Zhang, X.: New variants of a method of MRI scale standardization. IEEE TMI **19**(2), 143–150 (2000)
8. Otsu, N.: A threshold selection method from gray-level histograms. IEEE Trans. Syst. Man Cybern. (SMC) **9**(1), 62–66 (1979)
9. Ourselin, S., Roche, A., Prima, S., Ayache, N.: Block matching: a general framework to improve robustness of rigid registration of medical images. In: Delp, S.L., DiGoia, A.M., Jaramaz, B. (eds.) MICCAI 2000. LNCS, vol. 1935, pp. 557–566. Springer, Heidelberg (2000)
10. Smith, S.: Fast robust automated brain extraction. HBM **17**(3), 143–155 (2002)
11. Tustison, N., Avants, B., Cook, P., Zheng, Y., Egan, A., Yushkevich, P., Gee, J.: N4ITK: improved N3 bias correction. IEEE TMI **29**(6), 1310–1320 (2010)
12. Wang, L., Lai, H., Barker, G., Miller, D., Tofts, P.: Correction for variations in MRI scanner sensitivity in brain studies with histogram matching. MRM **39**(2), 322–327 (1998)
13. Weisenfeld, N., Warfield, S.: Normalization of joint image-intensity statistics in MRI using the Kullback-Leibler divergence. In: ISBI, pp. 101–104 (2004)

Spatial-Temporal Image-Constrained Lung 4D-CT Reconstruction for Radiotherapy Planning

Tiancheng He, Zhong Xue$^{(\boxtimes)}$, Nam Yu, Bin S. Teh,
and Stephen T. Wong

Houston Methodist Hospital, Houston Methodist Research Institute,
Weill Cornell Medical College, Houston, TX, USA
zxue@houstonmethodist.org

Abstract. Thoracic radiotherapy planning is increasingly dependent on 4D computed tomography (CT), which acquires axial images in multiple respirator phases and reconstructs them into 3D CT images based on respiratory signals. However, large reconstruction errors or artifacts may be observed due to poor reproducibility of breathing cycles. In this paper, 4D-CT reconstruction of helical mode CT scanning is achieved by incorporating spatial continuity and longitudinal smoothness of anatomical structures, such as chest surface, bone, vessel, and lung fields. The objective is to optimize the assignment of each axial image into different respiratory phases so that the artifacts or spatial disconti-nuity of anatomical structures are minimized, and the anatomical structures maintain their longitudinal consistency. In experiments, we compared our results visually and quantitatively with the current surrogate-based, image-matching-based, and chest surface-constrained methods. The results showed that the proposed algorithm yields better helical mode 4D-CT than other proposed methods.

Keywords: 4D-CT reconstruction · Respiratory motion · Registration · Bayesian model

1 Introduction

Radiotherapy is a traditional approach to treat lung cancer, and 4D-CT plays an important role on defining precise tumor margins. During planning, the clinical target volume (CTV) and planning target volume (PTV) are defined form 4D-CT to guarantee that PTV covers CTV, and normal tissues near the target are minimally damaged by the radiation dose. During radiotherapy, the planning 4D-CT images, the segmentation data, and radiation planning data are transformed automatically to the patient's onsite CT for treatment. 4D-CT acquisition obtains a large number of axial images in multiple respiratory phases and reconstructs a series of 3D-CT images to provide dynamic information of the lung and tumor. The efficient way to capture 4D-CT is either using cine mode or helical mode. In the cine mode, the axial images of different breathing cycles are captured at each table position, while the table is moving slowly and continuously when the scanning is being

© Springer International Publishing Switzerland 2014
M.G. Linguraru et al. (Eds.): CLIP 2014, LNCS 8680, pp. 126–133, 2014.
DOI: 10.1007/978-3-319-13909-8_16

performed in helical mode. Precisely reconstructing 4D-CT images is the key step to make sure that there is no topology artifacts both spatially and temporally in the image series.

In the literature, two categories of reconstruction methods have been studied. The first is using respiratory sensors, such as surrogate signals, spirometer, optical tracking, to record detailed breathing patterns [1]. All axial images with same breathing phase are sorted to reconstruct the 3D-CT images. The drawback is that some anatomical structures may be discontinued in the images [2–4] because the recorded signals are not always exactly periodical, and some axial images may be mis-grouped. The second category of methods tries to correct the reconstruction using image computing approaches, most of which are for 4D-CT reconstruction in the cine mode [5–8]. They could cause discontinuity of reconstructed images in helical mode because the different table position of each axial image is not considered. Recently, a Bayesian framework was proposed to reconstruct the helical 4D-CT using spatial and temporal smoothness constraints of the chest surfaces [9]. But the internal anatomical structures are not considered. In this paper, we extend the method [9] by considering the internal ana-tomical structures. The basic hypothesis is that anatomical structures such as lung field, vessels, and bones should have minimal spatial artifacts and have maximal temporal topology consistency.

The proposed Bayesian framework preserves the anatomical structures at each breathing phase by applying spatial continuity and temporal smoothness constraints, including chest surface, vessels, lung surface, and bones. An energy function is opti-mized by iteratively rearranging the axial images and optimizing the ideal anatomical structure constraints. After sorting, a non-uniform cubic B-Spline interpolation [10] is used for generating the final reconstructed images to deal with the unequal inter-slice distances.

In experiments, forty lung cancer patients undergoing radiotherapy planning were used to validate the proposed algorithm. The reconstructed results were compared with: (1) the external surrogate-based method, the default output from the Philips Pinnacle; (2) the slice-by-slice image matching-based method [7]; (3) the chest surface-con-strained reconstruction [9]. For visual comparison, the final reconstructed images were assessed by radiologists to count the mis-placed slices (artifacts). For quantitative comparison, the normalized spatial Boundary Shift Integral (BSI) [11] of anatomical structures from all the results was compared. Both results illustrated that our method outperformed other three methods, i.e., fewer artifacts form visual inspection, espe-cially at the region close to the diaphragm, and less sudden bumps of anatomical structures.

2 Method

When the axial images are captured in helical mode, the table of CT machine is set to move under a slow constant speed. This speed is determined by: (1) the setting of slice thickness, (2) respiratory cycle frequency, and (3) the number of simultaneously captured slices if the CT scanner has multiple row detectors. The goal is to cover the entire breathing cycle within a small table movement range. A synchronized surrogate signal is recorded during the scan. Using this signal, the axial images from each table position can be sorted to different breathing phases. The initial 3D images are formed from the sorted axial images. However, as mentioned previously, there are artifacts for the reconstructed images. Our proposed algorithm assesses such image assignment and corrects the mis-grouped ones based on the anatomical structure constraints. Given the current reconstructed serial 3D images, structures like lung field surface, chest surface, lung vessels, and bones are segmented, and longitudinal correspondences are calculated first by using deformable image registration. Then, spatial continuity and temporal smoothness of these anatomical structures will be applied in the optimization procedure to re-assess the assignment of each axial image.

Denoting the initial reconstructed serial images as $D = \{D_1, D_2, \ldots, D_K\}$, we can segment each image and obtain the serial segmented images $S = \{S_1, S_2, \ldots, S_K\}$. Each segmented image consists of a lung field surface L, a chest surface C, vessel structures V, and bone structure B, and $S_i = \{L_i, C_i, V_i, B_i\}$. K is the number of breathing phases. The objective for reconstruction is to assess the assignment of each axial image to form a new image sequence $I = \{I_1, I_2, \ldots, I_K\}$, and at the same time, the spatial continuity and temporal respiratory smoothness of the segmentation is guaranteed. To implement this idea, we use the formulation in [9] to jointly estimate the new serial images and a new ideal segmentation, denoted as $R_i = \{L'_i, C'_i, V'_i, B'_i\}, i = 1, 2, \ldots K$. The ideal segmentation represents how the anatomical structures should be. Using the Bayesian framework, I and R can be estimated by maximizing the following posteriori probability,

$$P(I, R|D) = P(D|I)P(I, R)/P(D) = P(D|I)P(I|R)P(R), \qquad (1)$$

where the initial images D is known, so $P(D) = 1$, and it is assumed that the ideal segmentation is independent form D. Using the Gibbs distribution for estimating the probabilities, we can use the following energy function to solve I and R:

$$E(I, R) = E(D|I) + \alpha E(I|R) + \beta E(R). \qquad (2)$$

α and β are the weighting factors. $E(D|I)$ denotes the degree of matching between the new serial image I and the initial data D, and it can be calculated by the normalized cross correlation-based similarity. $E(I|R)$ stands for the degree of matching between I and the ideal segmentation of anatomical structures R. Notice that S is the segmentation of I, so $E(I|R)$ is defined by a sum of distance between S and R,

$$E(I|R) = \text{dist}(S, R) = \sum_{i=1,\ldots,K} \text{d}\left(L_i, L'_i\right) + \text{d}\left(C_i, C'_i\right) + \text{d}\left(V_i, V'_i\right) + \text{d}\left(B_i, B'_i\right), \qquad (3)$$

where d() is the distance between the segmentations calculated according to [12]. For segmentation we use adaptive region growing extract the chest surfaces and bones, and used the segmentation method [13] to extract lung field surfaces and lung vessels.

The last term of Eq. (2), $E(R)$, represents the prior shape constraints of anatomical structures. Here, the spatial continuity and temporal smoothness constraints on R is applied. For spatial constraints, we only consider the continuity in z-direction because no in-plane axial image is altered. For temporal constraints, we make sure the temporal deformations applied on the segmented structures are smooth for neighboring respiratory phases. Thus, $E(R)$ is composed by two parts:

$$
E(R) = \frac{1}{K}\sum_{k=1}^{K} \frac{1}{|\Omega|} \left[\sum_x \left(\frac{\partial L_k^{'}(x)}{\partial z}\right)^2 + \sum_x \left(\frac{\partial C_k^{'}(x)}{\partial z}\right)^2 + \sum_x \left(\frac{\partial V_k^{'}(x)}{\partial z}\right)^2 + \sum_x \left(\frac{\partial B_k^{'}(x)}{\partial z}\right)^2 \right]
$$
$$
+ \lambda \frac{1}{K-1}\sum_{k=1}^{K-1} \frac{1}{|\Omega|} \sum_x \left\| \mathbf{f}_{k+1}(x + \mathbf{f}_k(x)) - \mathbf{f}_k(x)^2 \right\|,
$$

$$(4)$$

where λ is the tradeoff between spatial and temporal constraints, and Ω is the point set of R in phase k. The temporal deformation fields $\mathbf{f}_k, k = 1, \ldots, K-1$ are calculated by surface registration of R.

To minimize energy function in Eq. (2), we can alternatively calculate I and R. Given a series N axial images, we first sort them into K (typically 10) breathing phases according to collected surrogate signals, resulting image series D. Initially, we set $I = D$, and the minimization can be iteratively performed by (1) optimizing the ideal anatomical structures $R = \{L^{'}, C^{'}, V^{'}, B^{'}\}$ by fixing I, and (2) optimizing the image sequences I by fixing R. First, we segment image series I to get the segmentation result S, and R is initialized as S. Then, we apply registration to obtain the deformations $\mathbf{f}_k, k = 1, \ldots, K-1$. Finally, the ideal segmentation R can be updated using the finite gradient descent method:

$$
R \leftarrow R - \xi \frac{\alpha E(I|R) + \beta E(R)}{\partial R} \tag{5}
$$

where ξ is the updating step. After calculating R, we can calculate the updated 4D-CT image I. Basically, we iterate through all the axial images and re-assign each to the i th phase according to:

$$
i = \mathrm{argmin}_k (E(D|I) + \alpha E(I|R)). \tag{6}
$$

The optimization algorithm stops until the number of phase re-assignment is smaller than a prescribed number (5 in our case), and the algorithm generally stops after 3–4 iterations. It is worth noting that the major improvement of our algorithm over the chest surface-based reconstruction method is that all the major anatomical structures are considered during the image reconstruction. Our rationale is that the anatomical structures should maintain boundary continuity in the spatial domain, and their longitudinal motion (deformations) should also be smooth. Finally, after each axial image is assigned into their phase, the slices of each phase are arranged according to their table positions. For equaling the slice distances, we applied the non-uniform cubic B-Spline-based interpolation method [10] to resample them and reconstruct the 3D image sequences.

3   Results

In the experiments, we used datasets from forty patients undergoing radiation therapy of lung cancer by using Philips Pinnacle3 machine in helical mode. Each scan contains around 1400 slices. The thickness of each slice is 3.0 mm, and the resolution is 1.17 mm × 1.17 mm. According to the standard helical mode scanning procedure, the respiratory belt was used to monitor the breathing signals. The Pinnacle3 machine can perform initial 4D-CT reconstruction by using respiratory gating method. We used its reconstructed results as the initial input. Using the workstation with Microsoft Windows 7 professional, Intel i7 CPU (2.30 GHz), and 8.00 GB of RAM, our proposed algorithm was applied to refine the results, where α and β were selected as 0.5. We selected λ so that the weight of spatial smoothness is two folds to the weight of temporal smoothness.

Three other methods were performed for comparisons. The first is surrogate-based method the Pinnacle machine. After scanning, the Pinnacle3 machine will reconstruct the images according to the respiratory belt gating results. The second is the slice-by-slice image matching-based algorithm proposed by Carnes et al. [7]. In Carnes algorithm, the initial axial images are assigned into different respiratory phases manually. Then the slice-by-slice match method is used to sort the rest axial images. The image similarity measure for matching is normalized cross correlation. In our comparison, the sorting results of the first 20 axial images from the Pinnacle machine were used as the initialization for the Carnes algorithm. The third algorithm compared is the chest surface-based reconstruction method [9]. This method only uses the smoothness of chest surface as the constraints. For both the proposed method and the method in [9], we used the same initialization, i.e., the results of Pinnacle3 machine.

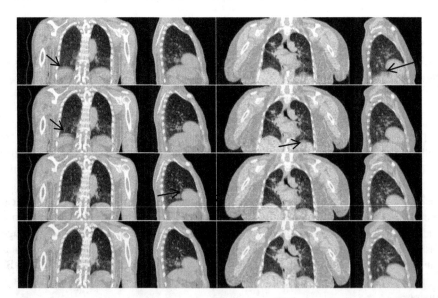

Fig. 1. Visual comparison of 4D-CT reconstruction results. First row: surrogate-based method; second row: Carnes algorithm; third row: chest surface-constrained method; and forth row: the proposed Bayesian 4D-CT reconstruction.

All results were visually assessed after reconstruction. Figure 1 illustrates the results from two different subjects. It can be seen that the artifacts from the results of surrogate-based method and Carnes algorithm are noticeable. The results on the third and the fourth rows are similar, although we can still notice some artifacts as pointed by the arrows. Overall, the proposed Bayesian 4D-CT reconstruction corrected the artifacts presented in other methods, and the anatomical structures in each 3D CT image look continuous.

For quantitative validation, the normalized spatial Boundary Shift Integral (BSI) [11] of the transition between the consequent reconstructed image slices was calculated. The BSI between two image slices for image I_k, $I_{k,i}$ and $I_{k,i+1}$, is defined as:

$$\beta_{k,i} = \frac{1}{(\alpha_H - \alpha_L)|\mathbb{R}|} \sum_{\mathbf{x} \in \mathbb{R}} \left[\text{clip}\left(I_{k,i}(\mathbf{x}), \alpha_L, \alpha_H\right) - \text{clip}(I_{k,i+1}(\mathbf{x}), \alpha_L, \alpha_H) \right], \quad (7)$$

where $\mathbb{R}$ is the set of voxels in the boundary regions of the segmentation R obtained using morphological operations. $|\mathbb{R}|$ is the number of voxels in $\mathbb{R}$. α_L and α_H ($\alpha_H > \alpha_L$) are the intensity range under consideration. In our experiment, we set $\alpha_H = 2500$, $\alpha_L = 0$ to cover CT values of all structures. The threshold function clip($\cdot$) is defined as:

$$\text{clip}(I, \alpha_L, \alpha_H) = \begin{cases} \alpha_L, & I(\mathbf{x}) < \alpha_L \\ I(\mathbf{x}), & \alpha_H \leq I(\mathbf{x}) \leq \alpha_H \\ \alpha_H, & I(\mathbf{x}) > \alpha_H \end{cases} . \quad (8)$$

Figure 2 shows the boxplots of the BSI values for all the 40 subjects. It is worth noting that lower BSI value means fewer artifacts in the image stacks of each 3D image for the subjects. Notice that the average BSI for an ideal 3D image without artifacts is not zero because the natural boundary shift exists in the image. In order to compare the quantitative results, we also calculated the average BSI from the breath-holding 3D CT images of the subjects. This allows for comparing the average BSI of 4D-CT reconstruction with the benchmark of real 3D CT images. From Fig. 2 it can be seen that the BSI values for the benchmark 3D CT images are the lowest among all the results, and the ones calculated from the reconstructed 4D-CT images using the proposed algorithm are very close to the benchmark values, reflecting much less artifacts generated from the serial 3D images.

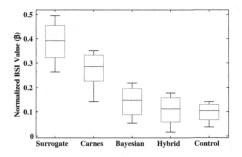

Fig. 2. Comparison of normalized spatial BSI.

To further evaluate the results, we plot the bone segmentation results of the reconstructed images. Figure 3 shows one example of the segmentation results, including the results using surrogate-based, image-matching-based, chest surface-based, and the proposed methods. Notice that the proposed method did not generate any obvious bone structure artifacts in the reconstructed image. On the other hand, some of the artifacts from other methods are visible and pointed out by red arrows. From visual and quantitative comparison, it can be concluded that less sudden jumps of anatomical structures were found using our method as compared to other methods based on the clinical datasets.

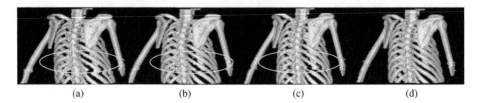

| (a) | (b) | (c) | (d) |

Fig. 3. Visualization of bones after image reconstruction. (a) Surrogate-based method; (b) Carnes algorithm; (c) chest surface-based reconstruction; (d) the proposed algorithm.

Further, two radiologists visually evaluated all the reconstructed results by counting the number of slices with artifacts, i.e., the slice with noticeable sudden jumps at anatomical structure. Figure 4 illustrates the box plots of such numbers of slices with artifacts. The results also confirmed the superiority of the proposed method as compared to others. Since it is difficult to give a further precise quantitative metrics due to the lack of ground truth, we will validate the quality using simulated 4D-CT images in the future.

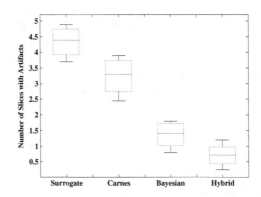

Fig. 4. Average numbers of evaluated artifact slices of 40 subjects.

4   Conclusion

We presented a Bayesian 4D-CT reconstruction algorithm for 4D CT reconstruction. Our rationale is that anatomical structures such as lung field, chest surface, bone, and lung vessels in the reconstructed images should preserve boundary continuity property either spatially or longitudinally. Using 40 clinical datasets for patients undergoing radiotherapy planning, the algorithm was compared with surrogate-based, image-matching-based, and chest surface-based algorithms. Both quantitative and qualitative comparison confirmed that the proposed algorithm outperformed the methods compared and yielded much less artifacts.

References

1. Lu, W., Parikh, P.J., Hubenschmidt, J.P., Bradley, J.D., Low, D.A.: A comparison between amplitude sorting and phase-angle sorting using external respiratory measurement for 4D CT. Med. Phys. **33**, 2964–2974 (2006)
2. Ehrhardt, J., Werner, R., Saring, D., Frenzel, T., Lu, W., Low, D., Handels, H.: An optical flow based method for improved reconstruction of 4D CT data sets acquired during free breathing. Med. Phys. **34**, 711–721 (2007)
3. Johnston, E., Diehn, M., Murphy, J.D., Loo Jr., B.W., Maxim, P.G.: Reducing 4D CT artifacts using optimized sorting based on anatomic similarity. Med. Phys. **38**, 2424–2429 (2011)
4. Han, D., Bayouth, J., Song, Q., Bhatia, S., Sonka, M., Wu, X.: Feature guided motion artifact reduction with structure-awareness in 4D CT images. In: IEEE Conference on Computer Vision and Pattern Recognition (CVPR), pp. 1057–1064. IEEE (2011)
5. Zeng, R., Fessler, J.A., Balter, J.M., Balter, P.A.: Iterative sorting for 4DCT images based on internal anatomy motion. In: 4th IEEE International Symposium on Biomedical Imaging, pp. 744–747. IEEE (2007)
6. Li, R., Lewis, J.H., Cervino, L.I., Jiang, S.B.: 4D CT sorting based on patient internal anatomy. Phys. Med. Biol. **54**, 4821–4833 (2009)
7. Carnes, G., Gaede, S., Yu, E., Van Dyk, J., Battista, J., Lee, T.Y.: A fully automated non-external marker 4D-CT sorting algorithm using a serial cine scanning protocol. Phys. Med. Biol. **54**, 2049–2066 (2009)
8. Gianoli, C., Riboldi, M., Spadea, M.F., Travaini, L.L., Ferrari, M., Mei, R., Orecchia, R., Baroni, G.: A multiple points method for 4D CT image sorting. Med. Phys. **38**, 656–667 (2011)
9. He, T., Xue, Z., Nitsch, P.L., Teh, B.S., Wong, S.T.: Helical mode lung 4D-CT reconstruction using bayesian model. In: Mori, K., Sakuma, I., Sato, Y., Barillot, C., Navab, N. (eds.) MICCAI 2013, Part III. LNCS, vol. 8151, pp. 33–40. Springer, Heidelberg (2013)
10. Neubert, A., Salvado, O., Acosta, O., Bourgeat, P., Fripp, J.: Constrained reverse diffusion for thick slice interpolation of 3D volumetric MRI images. Comput. Med. Imag. Graph. **36**, 130–138 (2012)
11. Freeborough, P.A., Fox, N.C.: The boundary shift integral: An accurate and robust measure of cerebral volume changes from registered repeat MRI. IEEE Trans. Med. Imag. **16**, 623–629 (1997)
12. Gerig, G., Jomier, M., Chakos, M.: Valmet: A new validation tool for assessing and improving 3D object segmentation. In: Niessen, W.J., Viergever, M.A. (eds.) MICCAI 2001. LNCS, vol. 2208, pp. 516–523. Springer, Heidelberg (2001)
13. Zhu, X., Xue, Z., Gao, X., Zhu, Y., Wong, S.T.C.: Voles: Vascularity-oriented level set algorithm for pulmonary vessel segmentation in image guided intervention therapy. In: IEEE International Symposium on Biomedical Imaging, pp. 1247–1250. IEEE Press, Boston (2009)

Simultaneous Multi-phase Coronary CT Angiography Analysis for Coronary Artery Disease Evaluation

Yechiel Lamash, Moti Freiman$^{(\boxtimes)}$, and Liran Goshen

Philips Healthcare, Haifa, Israel
{yechiel.lamash,moti.freiman}@philips.com

Abstract. Multi-Detector Computed Tomography (MDCT) is becoming increasingly important in the diagnosis of Coronary Artery Disease (CAD). Cardiac MDCT scan generally allows for reconstruction of several frames/phases in the cardiac cycle. The reconstructed images are then used to create curved multi-planar reformation (MPR) views wherein coronary lesions are best diagnosed. However, the generation of such MPR views for all potentially reconstructed phases is tedious and time consuming. Therefore, only a single phase is commonly used for diagnosis which may reduce the overall diagnostic accuracy. In the current work, we propose a new method that enable diagnosis of lesions from all reconstructed phases on a common MPR view simultaneously. Our method extracts the coronary centerline in one phase only. Next, it performs a fast registration of a region of interest between the multiple phases. Finally, the multiple phases are aligned to the MPR view and the clinician is able to review the multiple phases simultaneously. Our experiments indicate that the analysis time of multi-phase coronary CTA data can be reduced to less than 30 % of the currently required time using our method.

Keywords: Coronary CT angiography · Coronary artery disease · Multi-detector computed tomography · Registration

1 Introduction

Coronary artery disease (CAD), is one of the major causes for morbidity and mortality in the western world. Multi-Detector Computed Tomography (MDCT) is becoming increasingly important in the diagnosis of CAD. The diagnostic accuracy of cardiac CT data in assessing CAD is a major interest in the medical community since it may reduce the cost and risk of invasive coronary angiography [6].

One of the major challenges in cardiac CT imaging is handling the cardiac motion during the scan. The ECG signal is used to synchronize between the time domain and the heart's cyclic domain allowing the location of scan and reconstruction windows of a required heart phase. In general, cardiac scan is performed using two optional acquisition protocols: retrospective scan and prospective scan.

© Springer International Publishing Switzerland 2014
M.G. Linguraru et al. (Eds.): CLIP 2014, LNCS 8680, pp. 134–141, 2014.
DOI: 10.1007/978-3-319-13909-8_17

In retrospective scan, the reconstruction can be done in multiple phases all over the heart's cycle. In prospective scan, a prediction of the optimal mid-diastolic time point (phase 78 %) is performed slightly before the scan. The timing of the motion-free phase cannot be accurately predicted. Therefore, an over scan (phase tolerance) that allows the reconstruction of several phases is generally performed for the section of the optimal one. Commonly, the clinician reviews the axial slices to select the optimal phase.

However, lesions are best viewed in curved multi-planar reconstruction (MPR) images. The selection of a single optimal phase from several optional ones based on the review of axial slices has several limitations as follows:

- Since the lesions may appear in different spatial locations in the different phases due to its motion, the comparison of the phases' quality is sub-optimal.
- Phases' quality evaluated on the less effective axial slices rather than on MPR views which can provide more accurate visualization of the lesions.
- Generally the final diagnosis is performed on the selected phase rather than using all available phases.

These limitations may lead to sub-optimal diagnosis of CAD, especially in the case of soft-plaques which may appear as an artifact in a single phase.

Simultaneous multi-phase diagnosis holds the promise to straighten the certainty of clinical findings and to improve overall diagnostic accuracy of CAD using MDCT. However, the selection of the optimal phase by delineating or editing the coronaries' centerlines at each phase independently can be tedious and therefore impractical.

Several methods have been proposed for intra-phase alignment of the coronary arteries using landmarks [6], deformable model [8] and non-rigid registration [1,3]. However, these methods are not sufficiently robust and heavy in terms of computation time which prevents their utilization in the clinic. Recently Zuluaga et al. [9] proposed a local lesion registration method. While their method reduces the time required for navigation among different cardiac phases during the diagnosis process, it does not provide simultaneous multi-phase view for optimal diagnosis in the MPR view.

In this work we propose a new method and clinical workflow for simultaneous multi-phase MPR evaluation. First, the method generates the coronaries' centerlines on one phase using an automatic graph-based centerline extraction algorithm [5]. Next, the clinician indicates the region of interest to evaluate in multi-phase view. Next, the method performs a locally affine spatial re-synchronization across the multiple phases and projects the other phases' images onto the previously generated MPR view. Finally, the clinician can simultaneously evaluate the lesion in a spatially synchronized multi-phase view.

We demonstrated the benefit of the proposed method and workflow by comparing the time required to generate a simultaneous multi-phase view using our method to the time required with current workflow.

Our experiments show that the proposed workflow and method required less than 30 % of the time required by the current workflow.

2   Method

2.1   A Fast Simultaneous Multi-phase Coronary Analysis Workflow

The workflow stages are as follows:

1. The clinician uploads a single phase to cardiac application (for example phase 78 %).
2. The clinician runs coronary segmentation and centerline extraction to generate centerlines and MPR views of the coronary vessels in the current phase.
3. The user marks the suspected regions in the current phase MPR view.
4. The method spatially synchronized the regions of interest in the different phases to the current phase and projects thee data from the different phases onto the MRP view.
5. The clinician evaluates the lesions of interest in the different phases simultaneously.

We describe each computational step in detail next.

2.2   Coronary Centerline Extraction

We used the weighted shortest path methodology proposed by Freiman et al. [5] to compute the coronary centerline. The coronary centerline is defined as the shortest path between two graph nodes s and t corresponding to the coronary seed points. The CT image is described as a graph with edges connected adjunct voxels. The shortest path is the sequence of edges connecting s to t for which the sum of edge weights is minimized.

We defined the edge weighting function as a weighted sum of (1) the local intensity difference; (2) the seed deviation intensity difference; (3) the image gradient smoothness along the path; and (4) the path length:

$$
\begin{aligned}
W(x,y) =& \alpha \left(I(x) - I(y) \right)^2 \\
&+ \beta \left(\left(I(x) - I(s) \right)^2 + \left(I(x) - I(t) \right)^2 \right) \\
&+ \gamma | \cos^{-1} \left(\nabla I(x) \cdot \nabla I(y) \right) | + k
\end{aligned}
\tag{1}
$$

The first term is the squared difference between voxel x, y intensity values. This term penalizes for intensity differences along the path and prevents the path from leaving the vessel region. The second term is the sum of the relative squared differences of the seeds and edge-end voxel (y) intensity values. This term prevents the edges in the path from diverging from the intensity values of the user-defined seed points, and prevents the path from moving along locally smooth tissues with low edge weights instead of inside the noisy vessel. The third term is the angle between the intensity gradients along the path. This term ensures the smoothness of the image gradients along the path. The constant k is used to penalize long paths. The weighting constants α, β, γ are used to normalize the terms and to control the effect of each term on the overall path weight. Their values were determined experimentally and set once for all datasets. The shortest path is then computed using Dijkstra's algorithm [4].

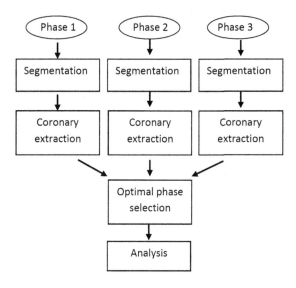

(a) Current Workflow

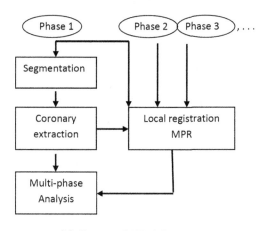

(b) Proposed Workflow

Fig. 1. Optimal phase selection workflow for multi-phase analysis. (a) current workflow, (b) proposed workflow.

2.3 Local Affine Registration

Since the relative motion of coronary vessels in adjacent phases is mainly translation with minor rotation and directional expansion, we assume that local affine registration [7] would be sufficient. Moreover, we would like the algorithm to run in real-time upon selection of object of interest (Fig. 1).

The registration functional is given by:

$$J = \sum_{\Omega} \left(I\left(W(x,p)\right) - T \right)^2 \tag{2}$$

I, T are the reference and template 3D images. To find a solution using the Gauss-Newton minimization scheme, we first develop the first-order Taylor expansion around p:

$$J(p + \triangle p) \approx \sum_{\Omega} \left(I\left(W(x,p)\right) + \nabla I \cdot \frac{\partial W}{\partial p} \triangle p - T \right)^2 \tag{3}$$

where ∇I is the image gradient warped to template coordinates, and $\frac{\partial W}{\partial p}$ is the Jacobian of the warp.

$$\frac{\partial J}{\partial \triangle p} = 2 \sum_{\Omega} \left[\nabla I \cdot \frac{\partial W}{\partial p} \right]^T \left[I(W(x,p)) + \nabla I \cdot \frac{\partial W}{\partial p} \triangle p - T \right] \tag{4}$$

Setting the expression to zero and solving yields the updated scheme:

$$\triangle p = -H^{-1} \cdot \left(\sum_{\Omega} \left[\nabla I \cdot \frac{\partial W}{\partial p} \right]^T \left[I(W(x,p)) - T \right] \right) \tag{5}$$

where H is the Gauss-Newton approximation to the Hessian:

$$H = \sum_{\Omega} \left[\nabla I \frac{\partial W}{\partial p} \right]^T \left[\nabla I \frac{\partial W}{\partial p} \right] \tag{6}$$

To improve the optimization runtime we used the inverse compositional update [2]:

$$\triangle p = H^{-1} \cdot \left(\sum_{\Omega} \left[\nabla T \cdot \frac{\partial W}{\partial p} \right]^T \left[I(W(x,p)) - T \right] \right) \tag{7}$$

where H is the Gauss-Newton approximation to the Hessian:

$$H = \sum_{\Omega} \left[\nabla T \frac{\partial W}{\partial p} \right]^T \left[\nabla T \frac{\partial W}{\partial p} \right] \tag{8}$$

The inverse compositional update scheme:

$$W(x;p) \leftarrow W(x;p) \circ W(x;\triangle p)^{-1} \tag{9}$$

The local affine registration algorithm is run in three course-to fine sub resolutions.

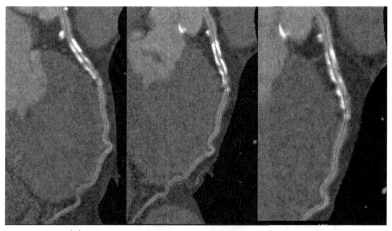

(a) Manual simultaneous multi-phase MPR view

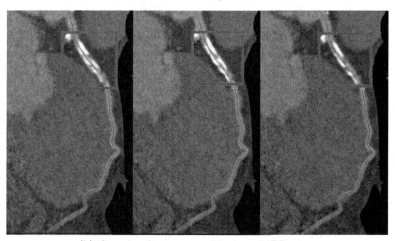

(b) Our simultaneous multi-phase MPR view

Fig. 2. (a) Three phases of the same coronary artery in MPR views. Each phase has a different centerline. Each phase image requires the overburden process of data uploading, segmentation and centerline editing or delineation. (b) The proposed approach: MPR views of coronary artery of phase 75 %. The blue marked region contains data of two other phases brought by image registration (Color figure online).

3   Experimental Results

We evaluated the reduction in time required to generate simultaneous multi-phase MPR view for CAD analysis by comparing existing workflow and our method. We took cardiac CT scans of seven patients from which four had retrospective scan and three had prospective scan. From the retrospective scans we

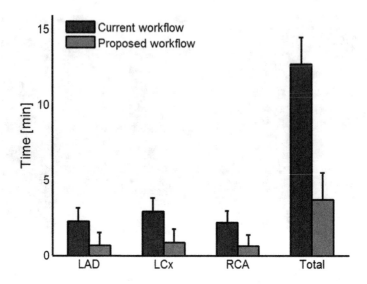

Fig. 3. Average and STD centerline editing times for the LAD, LCx, RCA and study's total time using the current workflow for optimal phase selection and using the proposed approach.

reconstructed two end-systolic phases and two mid-diastolic phases and from the prospective case we selected 3 mid-diastolic phases.

We generated simultaneous multi-phase MPR views for each patient by editing coronary centerlines for the Left Anterior Descending artery (LAD), Left Circumflex artery (LCx), and Right Coronary Artery (RCA) of each of the reconstructed phases independently using existing workflow. Next, we generated simultaneous multi-phase MPR views for each patient by delineating centerlines of the LAD, LCx and RCA on a single phase of the reconstructed phases and our method. Finally we compared the time required to generate the simultaneous multi-phase MPR views between the two methods.

Figure 2 presents representative example of the curved multi-planar images generated using the current workflow compared to the curved multi-planar images generated using the proposed workflow. We found that our proposed workflow and method reduced the time required to generate simultaneous multi-phase MPR views to less than 30 % of the currently required time. A detailed description of the required times depicted in Fig. 3.

4   Discussion and Conclusion

Improving the diagnostic accuracy of Coronary Artery Disease (CAD) using multi-detector cardiac CT data is a major interest for cardiologists and radiologists. The improved diagnostic accuracy of MDCT in assessing CAD has the potential to reduce the cost and risk of invasive angiography imaging. However, current workflow for cardiac CT evaluation is suboptimal and inefficient.

Coronary lesions such as plaque and calcifications are best seen in curved MPR views and in multiple phases. However, the time-consuming and tedious process required from the clinician to generate these views limited the current evaluation to a single phase which influenced the least by motion artifacts. The single view evaluation may yield to sub-optimal diagnosis. In the current study we reduces the time required to generate simultaneous multi-phase curved MPR views of the coronaries to less than 30 % of the time currently required to generate these multi-phase views. Our method and workflow first generate centerlines and curved MPR view on a single phase. Next, the user identifies lesions of interest and the algorithm register the rest of the phases to the current phase. Finally the other phases projected onto the curved MPR view to allow simultaneous evaluation of multi-phase data. This method hold the promise to improve overall coronary CT diagnostic accuracy by enabling simultaneous multi-phase evaluation of coronary CT in a clinically feasible time.

References

1. Aylward, S.R., Jomier, J., Weeks, S., Bullitt, E.: Registration and analysis of vascular images. Int. J. Comput. Vis. **55**(2–3), 123–138 (2003)
2. Baker, S., Matthews, I.: Lucas-kanade 20 years on: a unifying framework. Int. J. Comput. Vis. **56**(3), 221–255 (2004)
3. Chiu, A.M., Dey, D., Drangova, M., Boyd, W., Peters, T.M.: 3-d image guidance for minimally invasive robotic coronary artery bypass. Heart Surg. Forum **3**, 224–231 (2000). Forum Multimedia Publishing
4. Dijkstra, E.W.: A note on two problems in connexion with graphs. Numer. Math. **1**(1), 269–271 (1959)
5. Freiman, M., Joskowicz, L., Broide, N., Natanzon, M., Nammer, E., Shilon, O., Weizman, L., Sosna, J.: Carotid vasculature modeling from patient ct angiography studies for interventional procedures simulation. Int. J. Comput. Assist. Radiol. Surg. **7**(5), 799–812 (2012)
6. Harrington, R.A., Bates, E.R., Bridges, C.R., Eisenberg, M.J., Ferrari, V.A., Hlatky, M.A., Jacobs, A.K., Kaul, S., Moliterno, D.J., Mukherjee, D., et al.: Accf/acr/aha/nasci/saip/scai/scct 2010 expert consensus document on cardiovascular tomographic angiography. J. Am. Coll. Cardiol. **55**(23), 2663–2699 (2010)
7. Lucas, B.D., Kanade, T., et al.: An iterative image registration technique with an application to stereo vision. IJCAI **81**, 674–679 (1981)
8. Metz, C.T., et al.: Patient specific 4D coronary models from ECG-gated CTA data for intra-operative dynamic alignment of CTA with X-ray images. In: Yang, G.-Z., Hawkes, D., Rueckert, D., Noble, A., Taylor, C. (eds.) MICCAI 2009, Part I. LNCS, vol. 5761, pp. 369–376. Springer, Heidelberg (2009)
9. Zuluaga, M.A., Hoyos, M.H., Dávila, J.C., Uriza, L.F., Orkisz, M.: A fast lesion registration to assist coronary heart disease diagnosis in CTA images. In: Bolc, L., Tadeusiewicz, R., Chmielewski, L.J., Wojciechowski, K. (eds.) ICCVG 2012. LNCS, vol. 7594, pp. 710–717. Springer, Heidelberg (2012)

Ultrasound-Based Predication of Prostate Cancer in MRI-guided Biopsy

Nishant Uniyal[1], Farhad Imani[2], Amir Tahmasebi[3], Harsh Agarwal[3],
Shyam Bharat[3], Pingkun Yan[3], Jochen Kruecker[3], Jin Tae Kwak[4], Sheng Xu[4],
Bradford Wood[4], Peter Pinto[4], Baris Turkbey[4], Peter Choyke[4],
Purang Abolmaesumi[1], Parvin Mousavi[2], and Mehdi Moradi[1,5(✉)]

[1] University of British Columbia, Vancouver, BC, Canada
[2] Queen's University, Kingston, ON, Canada
[3] Philips Research North America, Briarcliff Manor, NY, USA
[4] National Institutes of Health, Bethesda, MD, USA
[5] IBM Almaden Research Center, San Jose, CA, USA
moradi@ece.ubc.ca

Abstract. In this paper, we report an *in vivo* clinical feasibility study for ultrasound-based detection of prostate cancer in MRI selected biopsy targets. *Methods*: Spectral analysis of a temporal sequence of ultrasound RF data reflected from a fixed location in the tissue results in features that can be used for separating cancerous from benign biopsies. Data from 18 biopsy cores and their respective histopathology are used in an innovative computational framework, consisting of unsupervised and supervised learning, to identify and verify cancer in regions as small as $1\,mm \times 1\,mm$. *Results*: In leave-one-subject-out cross validation experiments, an area under ROC of 0.91 is obtained for cancer detection in the biopsy cores. Cancer probability maps that highlight the predicted distribution of cancer along the biopsy core, also closely match histopathology. Our results demonstrate the potential of the RF time series to assist patient-specific targeting during prostate biopsy.

1 Introduction

Prostate cancer (PCa) is the most common type of solid tumor, and the second leading cause of cancer-related deaths in North American and European men. Early stage PCa, which represents the majority of cases diagnosed today, has many therapy options, including surgery, radiation therapy, brachytherapy, thermal ablation, and active surveillance. Selection of the optimal therapy and therapeutic dosage are chiefly determined by diagnosis and staging. Definitive diagnosis of PCa requires core needle biopsy, typically guided by transrectal ultrasound (TRUS). Current biopsy regimens involve systematic sampling of the prostate from eight or more predefined anatomical locations, followed by histopathological evaluation of these samples. The biopsy regimen is scaled to the

---

Nishant Uniyal and Farhad Imani: Joint first author

© Springer International Publishing Switzerland 2014
M.G. Linguraru et al. (Eds.): CLIP 2014, LNCS 8680, pp. 142–150, 2014.
DOI: 10.1007/978-3-319-13909-8_18

prostate gland based on its size and using nomograms but otherwise not tailored to the individual. TRUS-guided biopsy has rather poor sensitivity, with positive predictive values between 40–60 % [1]. Improved cancer yield can be achieved if patient-specific targeting is combined with systematic sampling. However, this is not feasible using TRUS alone.

In order to enable patient-specific targeting, other modes of ultrasound imaging such as radio frequency (RF) data analysis [2] and elastography [3] have been explored. These technologies, individually, have not entirely succeeded in accurate identification of high grade cancer.

Magnetic Resonance Imaging (MRI) has been used as an alternative modality to improve high grade PCa yield [4]. Guidelines for structured reporting of prostate cancer assessments based on multi-parametric MRI have been developed, involving simultaneous examination of T2-weighted, Dynamic Contrast Enhanced (DCE) T1-weighted, and Diffusion Weighted Imaging (DWI) sequences [5]. MRI-guided biopsy is, however, difficult, costly, time-consuming and not widespread. Fusion of ultrasound and MRI has been used to improve PCa detection by enabling targeting of the cancer foci pre-determined in MRI during TRUS-guided. Biopsy core locations determined in MRI are translated to patient coordinates using pre-procedure 3D TRUS and its registration to MRI [6]. 3D TRUS to MRI registration requires either sophisticated mechanical systems [7] to guide the biopsy needles or, if performed by software only [8], does not fully account for patient motion or organ deformation occurring during biopsy.

Recently, ultrasound RF time series, comprising a sequence of ultrasound RF frames captured in time from a stationary tissue location, has been used to effectively detect PCa in *ex vivo* and *in vivo* data [9]. In this paper, we propose to use ultrasound RF time series to complement MR-targeted biopsy procedures by providing cancer probability maps around MRI targets during biopsy. We envision that this solution should increase positive cancer yield in both MR-targeted and/or TRUS-guided biopsy procedures. It will also provide an opportunity to correct for mis-registrations of MR and TRUS images prior to sampling the tissue.

In the proposed solution, RF time series features have been used within an innovative computational framework that combines unsupervised clustering of the data with supervised classification. We use the histopathology of the biopsy cores for evaluation of cancer detection. Cancer probability maps are also shown, highlighting the distribution and the likelihood of cancerous tissue within the biopsy cores. In a single centre feasibility trial with data obtained from 14 subjects at 18 biopsy targets, we are able to predict the pathology of MRI-identified targets with high specificity and sensitivity.

2   Materials and Methods

2.1   Data Acquisition

Ultrasound RF time-series data is acquired on a Philips iU22 US scanner during MRI-guided targeted TRUS biopsies performed at National Institutes of Health

Clinical Center (NIH-CC), Bethesda, MD using the Philips UroNav platform. For targeted biopsy, pre-acquired T2-weighted MRI images are automatically fused with real-time TRUS images of the prostate [10]. Initially, the desired targets are delineated on the T2-weighted MRI image by a clinician based on the examination of four multi-parametric MR images: T2-weighted, DWI, DCE, and MR spectroscopy. At the beginning of the biopsy procedure, a series of electro-magnetically (EM) tracked 2D TRUS images of the prostate are acquired from base to apex. Next, a 3D US volume is reconstructed based on EM tracking data and registered to the MRI scan in the UroNav software. Following the registration of US and MR volumes, the targeted locations for biopsy are transformed to the EM coordinate frame. During the biopsy, the clinician navigates through the prostate volume to reach the desired target location for acquiring a core. Immediately prior to taking the biopsy, the clinician holds the TRUS transducer steady for 4–5 s to acquire RF time series data. Typically, 100 frames of RF time series data are acquired from each biopsy core. RF data is obtained prior to one, and in some cases, two biopsies of the MR-identified targets.

Ultrasound RF time series data is used from 18 biopsy cores of 14 subjects. Although RF time series data is collected in the axial plane, two biopsies are taken from axial and sagittal planes for each subject from the same location. The recording of the RF data and acquisition of the biopsy core are performed in sequence, not simultaneously, to avoid the appearance of the needle in the images. As a result, hand motion maybe present in some cases, between data and biopsy acquisition as well as during RF data recording. A quality control step is necessary to obtain a dataset with reliable reference label. In this step, we only choose to include subjects for which the histopathology of the axial and sagittal biopsies agree, and no excessive motion is present during RF time series acquisition. In our data, 10 biopsy cores are cancerous with Gleason scores above 6 and tumor areas $>40\%$. Eight biopsy cores are benign with consistent histopathological information.

2.2   Feature Extraction

Regions of Interest (ROIs): For each registered biopsy target, we analyze an area of 2 mm × 10 mm in the lateral and axial directions, respectively, along the projected needle path in the RF data, and centered on the target. The width of this area is close to the width of the biopsy core. The length of the biopsy core is typically larger than the 10 mm considered here; however, to account for mis-registration errors and possible hand-motions, we use a conservative estimate in this study. The selected 2 × 10 mm area is divided into 20 ROIs of size 1 × 1 mm resulting a total of 360 ROIs from all biopsy cores. For each ROI, we calculate the features described below.

Features: Nine tissue typing parameters are extracted using the spectral, fractal, and wavelet analysis of the RF time series data. Each RF time series contains 96 sequentially acquired frames of each RF sample of the imaging plane. We compute the spectrum of the zero-mean, hamming windowed, time series of an

RF sample and average the values over an ROI. Summation of the spectrum in four equally-spaced frequency bands constitute features 1–4 [11]. The intercept and slope of the fitted line to the spectrum in the entire frequency range are features 5 and 6. Fractal dimension of the time series is computed using Higuchi's method and averaged over an ROI as feature 7 [12]. We also calculate the central frequency (CF) of the spectrum as the mean of the spectrum bandwidth of the time series of an RF sample. The mean of the CF values (MCF) over an ROI is used as feature 8 [13]. Finally, we apply the discrete wavelet transform to the ultrasound RF time series of each RF sample using Daubechies 4 filter bank, where the signal is decomposed into approximation and detail coefficients at each decomposition level. The first approximation coefficient is computed for each RF sample in the imaging plane at the coarsest level (n = 3) of decomposition and averaged over each ROI as feature 9 [13].

2.3   The Proposed Classification Framework

Feature selection: Feature selection is performed using Recursive Feature Elimination (RFE), prior to classification to identify the optimal combination of the nine features described above for cancer detection. In this method, features are eliminated recursively based on their corresponding weight in a linear SVM classifier. Initially, the model is trained on all the features and their weights are calculated. Then, the feature with the smallest absolute weight value is eliminated. This process is repeated recursively; the number and combination of features resulting in the highest classification accuracy are used as the stopping criteria. In our case, the combination of two features resulted in the highest classification accuracy.

Classification: Even though our biopsy cores are assigned to cancer or benign pathologies, the selected tissue types are heterogeneous within these classes and could potentially be differentiated based on other structural differences. One approach to overcome "within class" differences is to first cluster the ROIs in an unsupervised manner. This could result in identifying the outliers of each class from the main distribution of the class. A cluster-specific classifier can then be used to differentiate cancerous and benign tissue in a supervised manner.

Experiments: We follow a leave-one-subject-out cross-validation strategy. Here, we train a classifier using the features extracted from the cancerous and benign ROIs of biopsy cores from 13 subjects and test on the features extracted from the ROIs of an unseen subject. In the first step of the process, ROIs from all 13 training subjects are clustered into two groups using k-means algorithm. Within each cluster, we train a Support Vector Machine (SVM) classifier to separate cancerous from benign ROIs. The next step constitutes testing, where we first assign the ROIs of the unseen subject to one of the clusters based on their Euclidean distances from the centroids of the clusters. The ROIs of the test subject are then classified using the classifier corresponding to their respective clusters. This process is repeated 14 times where every subject is left out for testing once. If in any of these leave-one-subject-out trials, a resulting cluster after the k-means step is over 90 % imbalanced (over 90 % benign or cancer), we do not train a classifier for that cluster and the label of test samples are determined based on majority voting in that cluster. In order to ensure that our process is not tailored to one type of classifier, we also use a Random Forests classifier and report our results using the two classification methods.

K-means clustering, SVM and Random Forests algorithms are implemented in the Scikit-learn machine learning package [14]. In addition to the binary class labels, we also generate the *a posteriori* class probability estimates for the biopsy core of each subject. The hyperparameters that need to be determined for the classifiers included the Radial Basis Function (RBF) exponent and the soft margin penalty coefficient for SVM, and the number and depth of the trees in the Random Forests. These are tuned using a grid search approach.

3   Results

The RFE feature selection process was repeated for every leave-one-subject-out experiment. It consistently isolated features 3 and 4 as the combination of features that result in the highest classification accuracy between cancerous versus benign tissue. These are both spectral parameters of the RF time series. Henceforth, we only use these two features in clustering and classification of the biopsy cores. Figure 1 shows the two clusters that are created by k-means for ROIs from all subjects. 190 out of 200 malignant ROIs are assigned to cluster 1 and 125 out of 160 benign ROIs are assigned to cluster 2. In other words, 95 % of all cancerous samples and 78 % of all benign samples are grouped in clusters 1 and 2, respectively. Based on this observation, and in order to maximize the number of training data per cluster, we limit the number of clusters to two.

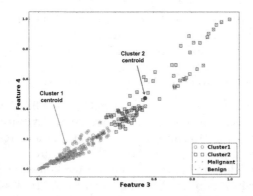

Fig. 1. Clustering performed on all 360 training samples.

The ROC curves are found in Fig. 2. The area under the curve is 0.91 and 0.90 for SVM and Random Forests methods, respectively. Colormaps that depict

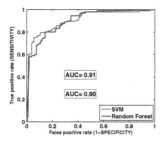

Fig. 2. ROC curves for SVM and Random Forests (each performed after clustering).

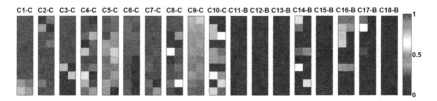

Fig. 3. Cancer probability colormaps of the 18 biopsy cores from 14 subjects with leave-one-subject-out cross validation using the best two RF time series features. Clustering and SVM classification is used.

the *a posteriori* cancer probabilities of ROIs in each of the 18 biopsy cores are illustrated in Fig. 3. The probability threshold to label an ROI cancerous in the cancer probability maps is chosen to be 0.6. It is noteworthy that if we eliminate the clustering step and perform classification with all training samples, we obtain an area under the curve of 0.88 and 0.89 for SVM and Random Forests methods, respectively.

Table 1 shows the percentage of the number of ROIs predicted as cancerous in each core, found in test samples in the leave-one-subject-out classification. The two different columns report the outcome for our method using SVM and Random Forests as classifiers. Using the SVM classifier, the percentage of cancer found in all benign cores is 45 % or smaller and in five out of eight benign subjects this number is zero. In the positive biopsy cores, we notice that the predicted percentage of cancer is above 60 % using the SVM classifier.

4   Discussion and Conclusion

We present a machine learning framework, consisting of supervised and unsupervised learning approaches, that uses RF time series analysis for the prediction of the histopathology of MR-guided targeted prostate biopsies. In a leave-one-subject-out study with data obtained from 18 biopsy cores in 14 subjects, we are able to accurately predict the pathology of MRI-identified targets with high specificity and sensitivity. In ROIs as small as 1 mm × 1 mm, and using only two spectral features of RF time series, an area under ROC curve of 0.91 is achieved.

Table 1. SVM and Random Forests cancer probabilities.

Subject	Biopsy Core	Biopsy Result	Gleason Score	Percentage of Cancer	
				SVM	Random Forests
1	Core 1	Adenocarcinoma	7	100 %	75 %
2	Core 2	Adenocarcinoma	8	90 %	85 %
	Core 3	Adenocarcinoma	8	70 %	70 %
3	Core 4	Adenocarcinoma	6	85 %	70 %
4	Core 5	Adenocarcinoma	9	95 %	95 %
	Core 6	Benign	0	45 %	25 %
5	Core 7	Adenocarcinoma	8	75 %	90 %
	Core 8	Adenocarcinoma	8	95 %	100 %
6	Core 9	Adenocarcinoma	7	75 %	70 %
7	Core 10	Adenocarcinoma	7	100 %	100 %
8	Core 11	Adenocarcinoma	7	60 %	70 %
9	Core 12	Benign	0	0 %	60 %
10	Core 13	Benign	0	0 %	0 %
11	Core 14	Benign	0	0 %	0 %
	Core 15	Benign	0	30 %	10 %
12	Core 16	Benign	0	0 %	0 %
13	Core 17	Benign	0	15 %	10 %
14	Core 18	Benign	0	0 %	0 %

Using k-means clustering, we show that these two features are able to separate cancerous and benign biopsy cores. Following classification, we calculate similar area under the ROC curve independently with SVM and Random Forests; this points to the stability of the proposed framework for tissue classification. We also present colormaps that depict the *a posteriori* cancer probabilities of ROIs in biopsy cores. These maps closely match the histopathology results of each biopsy core. As Table 1 shows, we report low cancer probabilities for all benign cores; specifically we predict zero probability for five out of eight benign cores. In other words, 63 % of the negative biopsies could have been avoided had we known the *a posteriori* cancer probability of that area using RF time series during biopsy. In terms of sensitivity, as is observed in Table 1, we report at least 60 % (mainly 70 % and up) cancer probability for all positive cores.

Our results demonstrate that RF time series can be used to complement MR-targeted biopsy procedures, by providing cancer probability maps around MRI targets during biopsy. Our proposed method could potentially increase positive cancer yield in both MR-targeted and/or TRUS-guided biopsy procedures. It could also be used to compensate for mis-registrations of MR and TRUS images prior to sampling the tissue for MRI guided prostate biopsies.

A limitation of our study is the size of the dataset. This is partly due to our conservative quality control step where we drop data from targets with conflicting pathology results in axial and sagittal planes. In addition, to minimize the impact of registration and targeting error on our analysis, we only choose ROIs in 10 mm length of the RF data centred around the target along the needle trajectory. A typical biopsy core could be as long as 18 mm. Data acquisition for a large clinical study is ongoing; the aim is to also incorporate a detailed histopathology reporting scheme where the direction of the cancer in a core is marked and results are reported in quarters along the biopsy core. We expect a larger dataset and more accurate mapping of histopathology to RF time series would further improve the results.

References

1. Rapiti, E., Schaffar, R., Iselin, C., Miralbell, R., Pelte, M.F., Weber, D., Zanetti, R., Neyroud-Caspar, I., Bouchardy, C.: Importance and determinants of Gleason score undergrading on biopsy sample of prostate cancer in a population-based study. BMC Urol. **13**(1), 19 (2013)
2. Feleppa, E., Porter, C., Ketterling, J.: Recent Advances in Ultrasonic Tissue-Type Imaging of the Prostate (2007)
3. Pallwein, L., Mitterberger, M., Struve, P., Pinggera, G., Horninger, W., Bartsch, G., Aigner, F., Lorenz, A., Pedross, F., Frauscher, F.: Real-time elastography for detecting prostate cancer: preliminary experience. BJU Int. **100**(1), 42–46 (2007)
4. Moradi, M., Salcudean, S.E., Chang, S.D., Jones, E.C., Buchan, N., Casey, R.G., Goldenberg, S.L., Kozlowski, P.: Multiparametric MRI maps for detection and grading of dominant prostate tumors. J. Magn. Reson. Imaging **35**(6), 1403–1413 (2012)
5. Barentsz, J.O., Richenberg, J., Clements, R., Choyke, P., Verma, S., Villeirs, G., Rouviere, O., Logager, V., Fütterer, J.J.: ESUR prostate MR guidelines 2012. Eur. Radiol. **22**(4), 746–757 (2012)
6. Natarajan, S., Marks, L.S., Margolis, D.J., Huang, J., Macairan, M.L., Lieu, P., Fenster, A.: Clinical application of a 3D ultrasound-guided prostate biopsy system. Urol. Oncol. **29**(3), 334–342 (2011)
7. Bax, J., Smith, D., Bartha, L., Montreuil, J., Sherebrin, S., Gardi, L., Edirisinghe, C., Fenster, A.: A compact mechatronic system for 3D ultrasound guided prostate interventions. Med. Phys. **38**(2), 1055 (2011)
8. Xu, S., Kruecker, J., Turkbey, B.: Real-time MRI-TRUS fusion for guidance of targeted prostate biopsies. Comput. Aided Surg. **13**(5), 255–264 (2008)
9. Moradi, M., Abolmaesumi, P., Siemens, D.R., Sauerbrei, E.E., Boag, A.H., Mousavi, P.: Augmenting detection of prostate cancer in transrectal ultrasound using SVM and RF time series. IEEE Trans. Biomed. Eng. **56**(9), 2214–2224 (2009)
10. Pinto, P., Chung, P., Rastinehad, A.: Ultrasound fusion guided prostate biopsy improves cancer detection following transrectal ultrasound biopsy and correlates with multiparametric magnetic resonance. J. Urol. **186**(4), 1281–1285 (2011)
11. Moradi, M., Mousavi, P., Siemens, D.R., Sauerbrei, E.E., Isotalo, P., Boag, A., Abolmaesumi, P.: Discrete Fourier analysis of ultrasound RF time series for detection of prostate cancer. In: IEEE EMBC, pp. 1339–1342 (2007)

12. Moradi, M., Abolmaesumi, P., Isotalo, P.A., Siemens, D.R., Sauerbrei, E.E., Mousavi, P.: Detection of prostate cancer from RF ultrasound echo signals using fractal analysis. In: IEEE EMBC, pp. 2400–2403 (2006)
13. Imani, F., et al.: Ultrasound-based characterization of prostate cancer: an *in vivo* clinical feasibility study. In: Mori, K., Sakuma, I., Sato, Y., Barillot, C., Navab, N. (eds.) MICCAI 2013, Part II. LNCS, vol. 8150, pp. 279–286. Springer, Heidelberg (2013)
14. Pedregosa, F., Varoquaux, G.: Scikit-learn: machine learning in Python. J. Mach. Learn. Res. **12**, 2825–2830 (2011)

Applying an Active Contour Model for Pre-operative Planning of Transapical Aortic Valve Replacement

Mustafa Bayraktar[1]($\boxtimes$), Bekir Sahin[2], Erol Yeniaras[3], and Kamran Iqbal[1]

[1] Department of Systems Engineering, UALR, Little Rock, AR 72204, USA
{mxbayraktar,kxiqbal}@ualr.edu
[2] Istanbul Technical University, Istanbul 34940, Turkey
bsahin@itu.edu.tr
[3] Halliburton, Houston, TX 77036, USA
yeniaraserol@halliburton.com

Abstract. Pre-operative plans for cardiac surgeries are required for providing precious information of the target area and assessing the suitability of offered interventional technique. This paper proposes a new approach to obtain the safest corridor along the left ventricle during pre-operative phase in order to register it onto intracardiac phase for transapical access. Method provides accurate spatial information of dynamic left ventricle borders by utilizing a modified active contour model during systole and diastole cycle of heart, and as a result of this, extracts the safest path through left ventricle based on magnetic resonance imaging (MRI) with promising volumetric capability and no-radiation effect.

Keywords: Pre-operative planning · Transapical access · Active contour model · Left ventricle border tracking

1 Introduction

Various operational techniques have been applied in heart valve surgeries since 1960s. Cardiopulmonary Bypass (CBP), which is the most conventional surgical technique, has been used for decades with adequate patient outcome [1]. In the early days, surgical access was gained via lateral thoracotomies; later median sternotomy was used as gateway to the heart. Throughout the world, this technique is widely used and performed even for patients from 80 to 90 years old [2]. Low ejection fraction, respiratory failure, cerebrovascular disease, pulmonary hypertension may develop at octogenarians and pose a risk for open heart surgeries. Regarding these constraints, search for a new technique has become a major issue in cardiac surgery. In mid 1990s, minimally invasive techniques started to emerge for cardiac surgeries. Compared to former, these techniques are more advantageous in terms of reducing skin, tissue and muscle damage [1]. For instance, Transapical Aortic

© Springer International Publishing Switzerland 2014
M.G. Linguraru et al. (Eds.): CLIP 2014, LNCS 8680, pp. 151–158, 2014.
DOI: 10.1007/978-3-319-13909-8_19

Valve Implantation (TA-AVI) is a new method for high risk patients with aortic valvular malfunctions, such as aortic stenosis or ejection insufficiency [3]. This technique has been performed on more than 30000 cases, showing that it will be an viable alternative to convenient surgeries [4]. One of the main functional advantages of TA-AVI is its ability to be applied on the beating heart, whereby CBP techniques as the name suggests take over the functionality of the heart and the lungs during surgery by a machine which sustains the oxygen and blood circulation. Regarding the risks of running body with the help of heart-lung machine, beating heart procedure technique is a revolutionary innovation. TA-AVI enables the placement of a stented bio-prosthetic valve through a left-lateral mini-invasion and the apex of the beating heart. When the delivery module reaches the correct position, the prosthesis is deployed by an inflatable balloon to pose in its final location [2,4]. In TA-AVI, once prosthesis is delivered, it cannot be repositioned again. This constraint increases the importance of appropriate positioning. Proper orientation avoids the coronary arteries that feed the heart muscles from obstruction, and mitral valve leaflets from damages.

- Pre-operative planning is a must for providing precious information about the target area in a procedure and means for evaluating stability and feasibility of the of-fered therapy technique. In TA-AVI, ejection fraction, cavity volume calculation, and safe path concepts are the basic elements of pre-operative planning. In this paper, we validated feasibility of Perona-Malik filtering aided active contours with-out edges based left ventricle border segmentation over determining the safest path for valve delivery module along left ventricle. Safe path determination is required from two aspects [5]. To reduce the surgery duration,
- To orient the delivery module safely along the left ventricular corridor without damaging the heart walls, mitral valve leaflets, and prevent potential adverse events during transapical access.

So far, a small number of approaches have been proposed to achieve preoperative planning for TA-AVI. Yeniaras et al. evaluated a method based on combining pre-operative multi-slice dynamic MRI with single-slice real-time MRI to update an access corridor from the apex to the aortic annulus [5]. Zhou et al. offered a Bayesian based algorithm to track landmarks of heart such as apex, medium, valve and centroid in long axis (LAX) and short axis (SAX) images [8]. However, both of them require user interaction and neglected volumetric assessment of left ventricle while contracting and expansion. These two works utilized MRI images, but did not take the papillary muscles into account, that drives the pre-operative planner trace the landmarks of left ventricle not accurately unless a robust segmentation method is used.

Addressing the challenges and weakness in the current approaches, we developed an approach that incorporates the novelties below:

- We propose to utilize Perona-Malik method as image filtering process before left ventricle border tracking has been initialized. Perona-Malik is a diffusion based method that helps us eliminate artifacts of papillary muscles on SAX MR images, while strictly keeping the edge information of left ventricle.

- Left ventricle border tracking step is based on a hybrid model which is combination of making a local region-based frame-work with the guidance of active con-tours without edges.
- In the last step, we calculated the means of x and y coordinate values of cropped segments and constructed 3D corridor by ordering each cropped contour on the z axis with 6 mm distance. Here, we should remark that 6 mm distance information is slice thickness and obtained from DICOM header of used MR images.
- The proposed algorithm can be run by single initialization, that is, localization of left ventricle by user, and the algorithm is propagated automatically to the other image slices acquired from their file location.

2   Imaging Session

A typical Cardiac Magnetic Resonance (CMR) examination consists of acquiring hundreds of SAX and LAX slices covering the whole cardiac-cycle. Manual segmentation of cardiac MR images is tedious and time-consuming; therefore automation and decreasing user interaction has become a necessity [2,9,10]. In our method, re-initialization for localization of left ventricle is not required, and the algorithm propagated over 325 SAX MR Images to build 3D model of the left ventricle. We validated the outcomes by comparing them to manual segmentation results, obtained by an experienced interpreter, which is considered as gold standard. Due to the low contrast structure and inhomogeneity of images examined, hybrid method is preferred to delineate the target area. The basic principle of the initiative is to divide local masks into two regions according to local intensity mean [5–7] (Fig. 1).

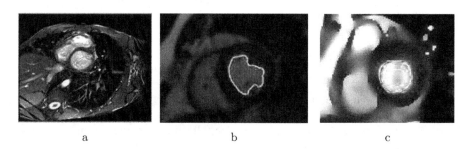

Fig. 1. (a) DICOM cardiac image; red circle represents the initial mask and the black color circle represents the local neighborhood. (b) Due to papillary muscles, segmentation cannot be achieved accurately. (c) Perona-Malik Anisotropic Diffusion eliminates papillary muscles artifact affects while keeping the edges (Color figure online)

Assume the black color circle at each point along the red color template. This circle is divided by the template (contour) into exterior and interior regions. The point is shown by the white dot. Black color circle represents the $V(x, y)$

neighborhood. Firstly, assume is a given image, C and is a closed contour as the zero level set of signed distance function and $C = x(x) = 0$. Interior of the contour C is shown by approximation of Heaviside function below.

$$\begin{cases} 1 & (x) < -\epsilon \\ 0 & (x) > -\epsilon \\ \frac{1}{2}\{1 + \frac{}{\epsilon} + \frac{1}{\pi}\sin(\frac{\pi(x)}{\epsilon})\} & \text{otherwise.} \end{cases} \quad (1)$$

A y point should be defined in addition to x, which is a planar variable and both represent a single point in the image domain (not the contour). A mask function $V(x, y)$ can be obtained from the distance between x and y with the respect to r, which is radius of the circle centered at x. Accordingly, if the distance between x and $y(x - y)$ is bigger than radius; function of $V(x, y)$ is equal to 0, otherwise is equal to 1 [7].

Per the information given above, the energy formula can be set as in Eq. 2.

$$E\vartheta = \int_{\Omega_x} \delta\vartheta(x) \int_{\Omega_y} V(x,y)F(I(y),\vartheta(y))dxdy. \quad (2)$$

In Eq. (2), F is a generic function that denotes local features at each point along the contour. On the other hand, energy function is obtained by the multiplication of a distance based function $V(x, y)$ and a force function.

Dirac function (x) forces the curve not to shift topology by evolving new contours randomly, while it lets the curve to split and merge. More explicitly, x points masked with $V(x, y)$ should be under (x) to confirm that F does not work on global statistics which are irrelevant to x [7]. After formulizing the energy outline, localization process is initialized by implanting local intensity means into energy outline. Local mean intensities can be calculated by multiplying mask function with global mean intensity. Approximations for global intensity mean can be represented as below;

$$j = \frac{\int_{\Omega_y} H\vartheta(y).I(y)dy}{\int_{\Omega_y} H\vartheta(y)dy} = \frac{\int_{\Omega_y}\left(1 - H\vartheta(y)\right).I(y)dy}{\int_{\Omega_y}\left(1 - H\vartheta(y)\right)dy}. \quad (3)$$

In Eq. (3) j and k denote interior and exterior regions, respectively. As expressed in [7], localized counterparts of j and k are computed by making use of $V(x, y)$ function, and are given in the following representation.

$$j = \frac{\int_{\Omega_y} V(x,y)H\vartheta(y).I(y)dy}{\int_{\Omega_y} V(x,y)H\vartheta(y)dy} = \frac{\int_{\Omega_y} V(x,y)\left(1 - H\vartheta(y)\right).I(y)dy}{\int_{\Omega_y} V(x,y)\left(1 - H\vartheta(y)\right)dy} \quad (4)$$

Local energies at each point along the contour can be calculated by j_l and k_l at each point along the contour. Hence, region-based energy term is given by the following *equation* [6,7];

$$E_L = \int_{\Omega} H\vartheta(y)(I(y) - j_1)^2 + (1 - (1 - H\varphi(y)))(I(y) - j_1)^2 dy. \quad (5)$$

Finally, a contour curvature term is added, given as, in order to keep the curve smooth. Thus, total energy formula can be defined as;

$$E(C) = E_L(C) + \lambda\eta. \tag{6}$$

where, weighting parameter is used for penalization of the arc lenght of the contour. Euler-Lagrange equations are used for minimizing energy equations with the purpose of obtaining contour evolution equations.

$$\frac{\partial\varphi}{\partial t} = \partial\vartheta - (\lambda\eta - (l - j_l)^2 + (l - k_1)^2). \tag{7}$$

The curvature smoother η can be computed as;

$$\eta = div\left(\frac{\triangledown\vartheta}{|\triangledown\vartheta|}\right). \tag{8}$$

j_l and k_l are kept updated until curve evolving ends. Simply, minimization can be performed if each point along the active contour has moved so that local statistics is best converged by local means j_l and k_l [7].

LV segmentation, which propagates the MR stacks, consists of these steps; 1. The initial contour is introduced, as a circle centered on the image with a reasonable radius. 2. Initialization of energy in terms of signed distance functions of. 3. Computing value by iteration process using the discrete form of curve evolution formula in (7). 4. Check, whether the solution is stable. If not, run f=f+1 again.

The discrete form of (6) can be approximated as $^{(f+1)} = \varphi^f + tU$ where U is the discrete form of energy minimization formula, which contains a weighting parameter λ that is generically set to 0.3. t is the time step-value used for enforcing stability and speed of curve evolution. The Courant-Freidrich-Lewy (CFL) condition which states that the numerical wave speed must be greater than the physical wave speed [6,7] is used for arranging mentioned constraints. The CFL condition can be represented as;

$$\triangledown < \frac{\triangledown}{max|U|}. \tag{9}$$

and CFL number usually lies between 0 and 1 to ensure stability [6]. It is a remarkable point that in order to increase the efficiency and speed up computation, initial value is updated in a narrow band around the zero level set but not on the whole image. Typically for MRI images ventricle cavity frontiers are measured to be 1.2 pixels wide for the narrow band width.

3   Experiments and Results

The utilized segmentation method has been applied 325 SAX MR Images acquired 2 health patients, who gave written informed consent. For each patient, a total of 25 images available at two time points; 13 slices at End Diastole and 12 slices are at End Systole. The comparison of the manual and automatic segmentation results over the left ventricle area and volume can give us idea regarding accuracy of our segmentation method. Table 1 displays the comparison of automatically computed left ventricle areas and volumes.

As can be seen in Fig. 2, cavity area decreases in the end-systolic frame. As mentioned in introduction chapter, aortic valve deformation causes aortic stenosis and aortic insufficiency (regurgitation), which are affections about blood ejection from LV to aorta. In the light of this clinical information, if the volume of transferred blood to aorta and remained blood in LV is assessed, i.e. to monitor the EF, the performance of the heart valve can be compared according to the standard value. In this work, LV volume information has been obtained and used for testing the accuracy of segmentation method.

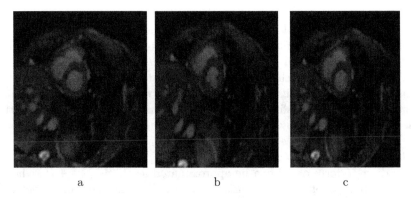

a   b   c

Fig. 2. (a)–(c): Diastolic to End-Systolic Left Ventricular Image Sequence. Contraction of left ventricle can be seen on the image sequence given in Fig. 2(a) through (c). The utilized segmentation algorithm propagates over slices and can track LV during heart cycles.

The cropped contours are concatenated in the three dimensional pixels coordinate system, xData and yData values are reachable in workspace menu of our software that uses pixel values in operations so that obtained result should be converted in actual values. Actual values of a DICOM MRI slice pixel can be retrieved by utilizing the software program's. Pixel Spacing values for x, y and Slice thickness for z value (for voxel). In addition to the slice thickness an inter-slice-gap that is %25–%50 of slice thickness has been added to z axis while volume calculation. For used images, these values are 1.25 mm, 1.25 mm, 6 mm, and 1.5 mm, respectively. Simpson rule is an accepted formula for left ventricular viable assessments. Simpson rule is represented as;

$$\sum_{i=0}^{t} 1 \ldots A_s.S_t. \tag{10}$$

In Eq. (10), t is the slice number, A is the area of slice and S is slice thickness or plus the slice gap. Simpson rule is based on classical volume calculation such as multiplication of the height with the area of a 3D object. According to the Simpson rule, summation of all elements of left ventricle surface area should be calculated, and multiplied with $1.25 * 1.25 * 7.5$, and divided by 1000 in order to convert the unit of result into centimeter cube.

Table 1. Area Comparison over the Left Ventricles (LV) of data sets between automatic and manual segmentation of cardiac MRI. Numbers represent ratio of automatic over manual segmentation results

	End Diastole	End Systole
LV Area Ratios	0.78	0.80
LV Volume Ratios	0.77	0.80

Safe path calculation is based on finding the center points of the segmented curves that represent the left ventricle boundaries. This can be done by considering the curve as a polygon and taking the center points of the values on x and y. In Fig. 3, safe path is visualized with a green color, and different thickness that implies the structure of the delivery module should be designed in the frame of information comes from the pre-operative planning, imaging part.

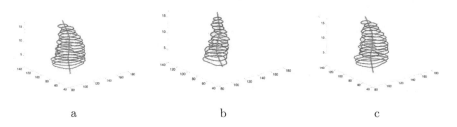

a   b   c

Fig. 3. Dynamic Safe Path Representation. Dynamic path is subject to change according to systole and diastole periods; (a) Represents End-Diastole Period (b) Represents End-Systole Period (c) Represents Transient Period between ED and ES Period

4 Conclusions

We introduced a novel computational pre-operative planning methodology for per-forming real-time TA-AVI in beating heart. Our study was dependent on generating a dynamic safe path and updating it on the fly, and the assessment of the anatomical structure of left ventricle. This work can be broadened with the process of registering the SAX segmented contours into LAX images to serve intraoperative cardiac procedures, and monitoring robotic module delivery application on the safest path.

References

1. Borger, M.A., et al.: Twenty-year results of the Hancock II bioprosthesis. J. Heart Valve Dis. **15**(1), 49–55 (2006)
2. Walther, T., et al., Transapical minimally invasive aortic valve implantation: the initial 50 patients. Eur J. Cardiothorac. Sur. Official J. Eur. Assoc. Cardiothorac. Sur, **33**(6), 983–998 (2008)
3. European Society of Cardiology, Cardiovascular Research and Nutrition, cardiovascular disesease. http://cardiovascres.oxfordjournals.org/content/73/2/253. full#ref-4
4. Yeniaras, E., Navkar, N.V., Sonmez, A.E., Shah, D.J., Deng, Z., Tsekos, N.V.: MR-based real time path planning for cardiac operations with transapical access. In: Fichtinger, G., Martel, A., Peters, T. (eds.) MICCAI 2011, Part I. LNCS, vol. 6891, pp. 25–32. Springer, Heidelberg (2011)
5. Chan, T.F., Vese, L.A.: Active contours without edges. IEEE Trans. Image Process. **10**(2), 266–277 (2001). (Citeseer)
6. Lankton, S., Tannenbaum, A.: Localizing region-based active contours. IEEE Trans. Image Process. **17**(11), 2029–2039 (2008)
7. Liu, J., et al.: Locally constrained active contour: a region-based level set for ovarian cancer metastasis segmentation. In: SPIE Medical Imaging (2014)
8. Zhou, Y., Yeniaras, E., Tsiamyrtzis, P., Tsekos, N., Pavlidis, I.: Collaborative tracking for MRI-guided robotic intervention on the beating heart. In: Jiang, T., Navab, N., Pluim, J.P.W., Viergever, M.A. (eds.) MICCAI 2010, Part III. LNCS, vol. 6363, pp. 351–358. Springer, Heidelberg (2010)
9. Uyanik, I., Lindner, P., Tsiamyrtzis, P., Shah, D., Tsekos, N.V., Pavlidis, I.T.: Applying a level set method for resolving physiologic motions in free-breathing and non-gated cardiac MRI. In: Ourselin, S., Rueckert, D., Smith, N. (eds.) FIMH 2013. LNCS, vol. 7945, pp. 466–473. Springer, Heidelberg (2013)
10. Bilgazyev, E., Uyanik, I., Unan, M., Shah, D., Tsekos, N.V., Leiss, E.L.: Using motion correction to improve real-time cardiac MRI reconstruction. In: Sixth International Conference on Machine Vision (ICMV 13), International Society for Optics and Photonics, pp. 90671I–90671I (2013)

Author Index

Printed in the United States
By Bookmasters